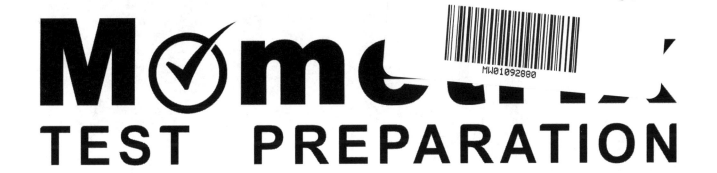

MLS

Exam Secrets
Study Guide
Part 2 of 2

DEAR FUTURE EXAM SUCCESS STORY

First of all, **THANK YOU** for purchasing Mometrix study materials!

Second, congratulations! You are one of the few determined test-takers who are committed to doing whatever it takes to excel on your exam. **You have come to the right place.** We developed these study materials with one goal in mind: to deliver you the information you need in a format that's concise and easy to use.

In addition to optimizing your guide for the content of the test, we've outlined our recommended steps for breaking down the preparation process into small, attainable goals so you can make sure you stay on track.

We've also analyzed the entire test-taking process, identifying the most common pitfalls and showing how you can overcome them and be ready for any curveball the test throws you.

Standardized testing is one of the biggest obstacles on your road to success, which only increases the importance of doing well in the high-pressure, high-stakes environment of test day. Your results on this test could have a significant impact on your future, and this guide provides the information and practical advice to help you achieve your full potential on test day.

Your success is our success

We would love to hear from you! If you would like to share the story of your exam success or if you have any questions or comments in regard to our products, please contact us at **800-673-8175** or **support@mometrix.com**.

Thanks again for your business and we wish you continued success!

Sincerely,
The Mometrix Test Preparation Team

> **Need more help? Check out our flashcards at:**
> **http://mometrixflashcards.com/MLSAMT**

TABLE OF CONTENTS

COAGULATION AND HEMOSTASIS _____ **1**
    GENERAL KNOWLEDGE _____ 1
    COAGULATION PROCEDURES _____ 5

IMMUNOLOGY AND SEROLOGY _____ **10**
    GENERAL KNOWLEDGE _____ 10
    SEROLOGICAL TESTS FOR SYPHILIS _____ 12
    ANALYTICAL PROCEDURES _____ 13
    SPECIAL PROCEDURES_____ 16

IMMUNOHEMATOLOGY_____ **17**
    GENERAL KNOWLEDGE _____ 17
    BLOOD TYPING _____ 20
    IMMUNE RESPONSE _____ 23
    COMPATIBILITY TESTING_____ 31
    RH IMMUNE GLOBULIN _____ 33
    SPECIAL TESTS_____ 34

BLOOD BANKING AND TRANSFUSION SERVICES _____ **36**
    GENERAL KNOWLEDGE _____ 36
    BLOOD BANKING PRACTICES _____ 50

MICROBIOLOGY_____ **52**
    GENERAL KNOWLEDGE _____ 52
    MEDIA QUALITY CONTROL, TECHNIQUES, AND CULTURES_____ 56
    BACTERIAL IDENTIFICATION _____ 65
    SPECIAL TESTS_____ 71
    VIROLOGY _____ 74
    PARASITOLOGY_____ 76
    MYCOLOGY _____ 79

URINALYSIS AND BODY FLUIDS_____ **84**
    GENERAL KNOWLEDGE _____ 84
    URINALYSIS PROCEDURES _____ 85
    SPECIAL TESTS_____ 89

PRACTICE TEST _____ **92**

ANSWER KEY AND EXPLANATIONS _____ **99**
    ANSWER EXPLANATIONS_____ 100

HOW TO OVERCOME TEST ANXIETY _____ **108**

ADDITIONAL BONUS MATERIAL _____ **114**

Coagulation and Hemostasis

General Knowledge

HEMOSTASIS

Hemostasis is the cessation of bleeding. There are four main steps involved in hemostasis: 1. A damaged blood vessel narrows (vasoconstriction) and the reduced diameter helps slow down any bleeding. 2. Platelets that are present in the blood attach themselves to the collagen in the walls of the blood vessel to create a hemostatic plug within seconds. This process is sometimes referred to as primary hemostasis. After the formation of a hemostatic plug, secondary hemostasis occurs. The clotting factors help fibrin form from fibrinogen. The fibrin then aids in the formation of blood clot at the wound site. Secondary hemostasis takes a few minutes. 3. The newly-formed blood clot helps the wound site create new smooth muscle cells to repair the wound. The clot can then be lyzed (destroyed) when it is not needed any longer.

COAGULATION TERMINOLOGY

Coagulation	Formation of a clot. Four stage process: (1) Damaged vessel constricts (2) Platelets adhere to damaged area (platelet adhesion) to form a platelet plug (3) Extrinsic and intrinsic pathways lead to common pathway in which prothrombin activator reacts with calcium ions to form prothrombin, which forms thrombin, which causes fibrinogen to form fibrin monomers that react with fibrin stabilizing factor and calcium ions to form fibrin polymers that attract platelets and phospholipids to form a clot (4) Fibrinolysis (clot breakdown) occurs when plasmin breaks fibrin into fragments, which are then removed by phagocytes
Sodium citrate	Sodium citrate is an anticoagulant (crystalline compound) that prevents clotting but preserves coagulation factors.
Thrombin	Clot activator that converts fibrinogen into fibrin.
Platelet function test	Platelet function tests assess the ability of platelets to form a clot and help to diagnose bleeding disorders.
Warfarin (Coumadin®)	Warfarin (Coumadin®) is an anticoagulant that interferes with the formation of vitamin K–associated clotting factors (II, VII, IX, X) and C and S anticoagulant proteins.
Fibrin	Fibrin is a protein that aids in blood clotting. Along with platelets, fibrin helps form blood clots. Fibrin is made from the glycoprotein fibrinogen, in the liver.
Heparin	Heparin is a polysaccharide anticoagulant that helps prevent blood clotting. Heparin is concentrated in the vessels surrounding the liver and the lungs. It can also be found in the spleen and various other muscles. Heparin is also a drug that can be given to patients that need to take advantage of its anticoagulant properties, such as in the case of a pulmonary embolism.
Plasmin	Plasmin is an enzyme that helps dissolve (lyze) fibrin that is present in blood clots. Lyzing a clot turns coagulated blood into liquid blood again. Plasmin is derived from plasminogen in the blood plasma.

1

FUNCTIONS OF COAGULATION FACTORS

Coagulation factors, along with plasma proteins, tissues, and calcium, work with one another on the surface of platelets to form fibrin clots. A cascade must be followed through these factors and mechanisms properly for adequate clot formation. Listed below are the coagulation factors and their functions in the coagulation cascade:

Factor	Name	Function
I	Fibrinogen	Forms clots
II	Prothrombin	Activates I, I, VII, VIII, XI, XIII, protein C, and platelets
III	Tissue factor	Cofactor of VIIa
IV	Ionized calcium	Needed for factors to bind to phospholipids
V	Labile factor	Cofactor of X; forms the prothrombinase complex
VII	Stable factor	Activates IX and X
VIII:C	AHF	Cofactor of IX; forms tenase complex
VIII:vWF	von Willebrand factor (vWF)	Cofactor; accelerates enzymatic reactions
IX	Plasma thromboplastin component	Activates X; forms a tenase complex with VIII
X	Stuart–Prower factor	Activates II; forms a prothrombinase complex with V
XI	Plasma thromboplastin antecedent	Activates IX
XII	Hageman factor	Activates XI, VII, PK, and plasminogen
XIII	Fibrin-stabilizing factor	Crosslinks fibrin
PK	Prekallikrein	Activates XII and PK; cleaves HMWK
HMWK	High-molecular-weight kininogen	Supports activation of XII, XI, and PK

HEMOPHILIA

Hemophilia is an inherited disease in which the body has trouble forming blood clots because it lacks a clotting factor. People afflicted with hemophilia have the tendency to hemorrhage and have episodes of uncontrolled bleeding. The bleeding can either be external or internal. Hemophilia is a sex-linked disease (recessive on the X chromosome), and because of this, males are more likely to be hemophiliacs than are females. Many royal families in Europe inherited hemophilia from Queen Victoria. Hemophilia is passed from mother (the carrier) to son. There are three types of hemophilia, A, B, and C. These types are all defined by a different deficiency in a clotting factor necessary for the formation of blood clots and for the control of bleeding.

ADJUSTING ANTICOAGULANT-TO-BLOOD RATIO

Anticoagulant-blood ratio adjustment: If a patient's hematocrit is higher than 55%, it is more viscous than normal and contains a lower percentage of plasma. Because of this, for samples collected in a tube with anticoagulant, such as sodium citrate, centrifugation will result in plasma with an increased level of anticoagulant. This, in turn, can affect the test results for all tests run on the sample, so a second sample with anticoagulant corrected should be obtained. For example, a formula is applied to determine the amount of sodium citrate to remove from a tube. For calculation, a 5-mL tube contains 4.5 mL of blood; a 3-mL tube, 2.7 mL; and a 2 mL, 1.8 mL. The volume of sodium citrate for 5-mL tube is 0.5 mL, for the 3-mL tube is 0.3 mL, and for the 2-mL tube is 0.2 mL:

$$Sodium\ citrate\ volume = (1.85 \times 10^{-3}) \times (100 - HCT) \times (blood\ volume)$$

Once the volume needed is determined, then the excess anticoagulant is removed from the tube before the blood draw. Correction charts are also available for the various tube sizes. For 5 mL (4.5 mL) tube:

Hematocrit	Sodium citrate volume
57	0.36 mL
63	0.31 mL

FIBRINOLYSIS AND COAGULATION INHIBITORS AND EFFECT OF HEPARIN

Alpha 2-antiplasmin: inhibits fibrinolysis; not affected by heparin

Alpha 1-antitrypsin: alters coagulation factor XI; not affected by heparin

Alpha 2-macroglobulin: alters the function and development of plasmin; not affected by heparin

Antithrombin III: obstructs the function of factors IX, X, XI, XII, plasmin, and kallikrein; made more effective by heparin

C1 inactivator: obstructs the function of factors XI, XII, and plasmin; not affected by heparin

PLATELET COAGULATION GROUPS

Contact group: contains the coagulation factors XI, XII, high molecular weight kininogen, and prekallikrein; all of these factors are created in the liver and serve to activate fibrinolysis, intrinsic coagulation activation, and the activation of the complement system

Prothrombin group: contains coagulation factors II, VII, IX, and X; these factors are produced in the liver and require vitamin K; anticoagulation therapies and antibiotics may decrease the activity of these coagulation factors

Fibrinogen group: contains coagulation factors I, V, VIII, and XIII; these factors do not require vitamin K, and, with the exception of factor VIII, are located in platelets; these factors are substrates for the fibrinolytic enzyme plasmin

HYPERCOAGULABILITY ASSESSMENT

Hypercoagulability is described as a condition in which blood has a higher tendency to clot and cause thrombosis. Hypercoagulable states can be hereditary, that is, caused by abnormal protein activity and anticoagulant antibodies, or they can be acquired, for example, due to reactions to anticoagulant medications. Various laboratory assays are performed to determine the cause of hypercoagulability.

Lupus anticoagulant and **antiphospholipid antibodies** are indicated by prolonged PT and APTT results and require further assessment. Mixing studies are performed to verify the presence of an inhibitor, including the lupus anticoagulant and to confirm antiphospholipid dependency. Lupus anticoagulant antibodies are quantified using the Bethesda assay, by adding normal plasma to the sample and incubating the mixtures at 37 °C. The amount of normal plasma required to neutralize the lupus anticoagulant is directly proportional to the amount of antibody present in the sample.

TYPES OF HEMOPHILIA

Hemophilia A is also referred to as "classic hemophilia". This is the most common form of hemophilia, and it is due to a deficiency in Factor VIII. Females are carriers. This disease affects males and leads to a prolonged clotting time and bleeding episodes. Less than 10 IU of factor VIII is characteristic of hemophilia A. Hemophilia A is 7 times more prevalent than Hemophilia B (Christmas disease), a deficiency or mutation of Factor IX. Christmas disease is also X-linked, and affects mostly males. People with Hemophilia B are at increased risk of hemorrhage. Finally, Hemophilia C is identified by the deficiency of Factor XI. This disease affects both sexes, and is an autosomal recessive disorder affecting primarily Jews of Ashkenazi descent. People with Hemophilia C often do not require treatment, and the disease is usually not severe. There is also no bleeding at the joints, as seen with Hemophilia A and B.

BERNARD-SOULIER SYNDROME

Bernard-Soulier syndrome is a disease that is due to the lack of glycoprotein Ib, which is normally present in the membranes of platelets. Glycoprotein Ib is the protein that reacts with the von Willebrand factor, and its absence causes problems in platelet aggregation and in the forming of blood clots. Platelets in a person with Bernard-Soulier syndrome are larger and more spherical than normal platelets, and their membranes are not as strong. This disease is inherited, and affects both males and females with an equal frequency.

CHRISTMAS DISEASE

Christmas disease is an inherited, X-chromosome linked disease affecting only males (because of their XY phenotype). Females are carriers. Christmas disease is characterized by the lack of clotting Factor IX, a protein that is normally found in plasma, necessary for platelet aggregation and the formation of blood clots. Without Factor IX, a patient is more likely to experience hemorrhage when injured, and abnormal bleeding episodes like nosebleeds, bruising, joint swelling, hematuria, hematochezia and melena. Christmas disease is sometimes called Hemophilia B. It is treated with regular injections of Factor IX. Classical Hemophilia A is treated with Factor VIII.

VON WILLEBRAND'S DISEASE

Von Willebrand's disease is a hereditary defect on Chromosome 12 that causes the von Willebrand factor, necessary for clotting, to either be absent or defective. Unlike Hemophilia A and B, both females and males can have von Willebrand's disease, and it especially targets people with blood type O. The von Willebrand factor (vWF) is a protein that aids in platelet aggregation and blood clotting, and it helps control platelet activity. Without the von Willebrand factor, or with a deficient factor, patients have menorrhagia (heavy menstruation), epistaxis (nosebleeds), and bruising. Type I and II cases of von Willebrand's disease are mild and require no treatment, except when patients are undergoing surgery or dental work. Type III is severe, with spontaneous bleeding into their joints. Patients use Demoprexin, Cyklokapron, Amicar, and thrombin powder on cuts to control bleeding.

MOLECULAR TESTING AND MOLECULAR ASSAYS IN COAGULATION

Molecular testing and molecular assays are used in coagulation studies because they have increased specificity as well as increased sensitivity, and testing can be carried out while the patient is receiving anticoagulant medications. Molecular testing is especially useful for inherited diseases because many coagulation disorders (factor V Leiden mutation, hyperhomocysteinemia, and prothrombin 20210 G>A mutation) and bleeding disorders (hemophilia A and B, von Willebrand disease) involve molecular defects. However, in some cases molecular testing is not practical because of numerous possible mutations, such as with antithrombin testing and protein C and S deficiencies. Numerous different types of procedure are utilized, but one of the most common is the PCR-based assay, especially for inherited clotting disorders, with restriction fragment length polymorphism analysis or other methods. A number of direct hybridization methods, such as the Invader assay, are also available.

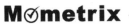

HEPARIN NEUTRALIZATION

Patient samples with unexpectedly prolonged APTT results should be investigated for heparin contamination. Contaminated samples exhibit reduced platelet function and increased clotting times due to the medication's anticoagulant nature. APTT samples may be collected from an IV after heparin administration; however, the tubing must be appropriately flushed with saline and 10 mL of blood must be collected and discarded prior to sample collection. Failure to properly flush an IV or discard blood prior to collection leads to heparin neutralization. Heparin neutralization occurs in patients not receiving anticoagulants by contamination of the sample tube during collection or filling it with blood from another tube containing heparin. The bacterial enzyme heparinase is added to 1 mL of platelet-poor plasma to confirm or deny the suspicion of heparin contamination in a sample. Heparinase degrades unfractionated and low-molecular-weight heparin by cleaving their molecules at multiple binding sites and reducing anticoagulation properties. A normal APTT result following the addition of heparinase, and a 15-minute incubation at room temperature confirms contamination by the presence of up to 2 units/mL of heparin in a sample.

Coagulation Procedures

Prothrombin time (PT)	10–14 seconds	Collect 1 mL blood in sodium citrate blue-capped tube (completely filled).
		Increased: Anticoagulation therapy, vitamin K deficiency, decreased prothrombin, DIC, liver disease, and malignant neoplasm. Some drugs may shorten time.
Partial thromboplastin time (PTT)	30–45 seconds	Collect 1 mL blood in sodium citrate blue-capped tube (completely filled).
		Increased: Hemophilia A & B, von Willebrand disease, vitamin deficiency, lupus, DIC, and liver disease
Activated partial thromboplastin time (aPTT)	21–35 seconds	Collect 1 mL blood in sodium citrate blue-capped tube (completely filled).
		Similar to PTT but an activator added that speeds clotting time. Used to monitor heparin dosage. Increased: Hemophilia A & B, von Willebrand disease, vitamin deficiency, lupus, DIC, and liver disease Decreased: Extensive cancer, early DIC, and after acute hemorrhage
D-dimer	0.5 mcg/mL FEU*	Collect 1 mL blood in sodium citrate blue-capped tube (completely filled) for immunoturbidimetry. Transport frozen.
		D-dimer is a specific polymer that results when fibrin breaks down, giving a marker to indicate the degree of fibrinolysis. Increased: DIC, pulmonary embolism, DVT, late pregnancy, neoplastic disorder, preeclampsia, arterial/venous thrombosis
Fibrinogen (Factor I)	100-400 mg/dL	Collect 1 mL blood in sodium citrate blue-capped tube (completely filled) for photo-optical clot detection.

5

		Synthesized in liver, converts to fibrin, which combines with platelets in coagulation sequence. Increased: Acute MI, cancer, eclampsia, multiple myeloma, Hodgkin's disease, nephrotic syndrome, tissue trauma Decreased: DIC, liver disease, congenital fibrinogen abnormality
Fibrin degradation product (fibrin split products [FSPs])	<5 mcg/mL FEU*	Collect 1 mL blood in sodium citrate blue-capped tube (completely filled) for latex agglutination test. Transport frozen.
		FSPs occur as clots form and more breakdown of fibrinogen and fibrin occurs, interfering with blood coagulation by coating platelets and disrupting thrombin, and attaching to fibrinogen so stable clots can't form. Increased: DIC, liver disease, MI, hemorrhage, pulmonary embolism, renal disease, obstetric complications, kidney transplant rejection
Heparin assay (Antithrombin III)	1-3 mo: 48-108%	Collect 1 mL blood in sodium citrate blue-capped tube (completely filled) for chromogenic immunoturbidimetry.
	1-5 y: 82-139%	Utilized to diagnose heparin resistance in patients receiving heparin therapy and to diagnose hypercoagulable conditions.
	6-17 y: 90-131%	
		Increased: Acute hepatitis, kidney transplantation, vitamin K deficiency
	>18 y: 80-120%	Decreased: DIC, liver transplantation, nephrotic syndrome, pulmonary embolism, venous thrombosis, liver failure, cirrhosis, carcinoma
Platelet aggregation	Results vary according to laboratory.	Collect 4-5 mL sample in sodium citrate tubes for analysis with light transmission aggregometer. Must be processed within 60 minutes of collection.
		Test measures the ability of platelets to aggregate and form clots in response to various activators. Decreased: Myeloproliferative disorders, autoimmune disorders, uremia, clotting disorders, and adverse effects of medications. Drugs that affect clotting should be avoided before test for up to 2 weeks (on advice of physician).

FEU* = fibrinogen equivalent units

MIXING STUDIES AND FACTOR TESTING

Mixing studies are used to determine if abnormal test results for the PT and/or aPTT are because of coagulation deficiency or because of factor inhibitors. Because normal results still occur when PT and aPTT levels are at 50%, the test involves mixing equal amounts of the patient's plasma with a sample of plasma in which the coagulation factors are normal (leading to a 50% level). If the abnormal findings resulted from deficiency, the PT and aPTT results will be within normal range, but if the abnormal findings resulted from inhibitors, then the clotting times will be prolonged.

Factor testing is usually done when the PT and aPTT are abnormally prolonged (or in some cases for thrombosis) to determine the presence and type of clotting abnormality. Factor levels vary, so

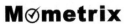

factor testing generally reports factors as a percentage of normal (which is 100%). Low percentages indicate hypocoagulopathy and percentages above 100% indicate hypercoagulopathy.

FACTOR ASSAYS

Factor assays are functional clotting assays performed to confirm a deficiency of one or more coagulation factors. Patient plasma is added to factor-deficient reagent plasma in 1:10, 1:20, and 1:40 dilutions, and the prothrombin time (PT) or activated prothrombin time (APTT) of each dilution is measured. Results obtained for each sample dilution are plotted on a line graph and compared to a standard curve to assess the activity of a specific factor. The amount of correction to the PT or APTT clotting time in diluted samples is indicative of the activity of the factor being studied. The activity of factors V, VII, X, and II is determined via PT-based assays, whereas that of factors VIII, IX, XI, and XII is measured with APTT-based assays. Russell's viper venom (RVV) factor assays are performed to determine a deficiency in factor X. The RVV factor assay comprises a series of dilutions of factor-deficient plasma incubated at 37 °C for 30 seconds with the addition of RVV and calcium chloride. The time it takes for a clot to form is recorded and compared to a standard curve to establish factor X activity.

ISSUES WITH COAGUALTION INHIBITORS

Natural coagulation inhibitors circulate in the bloodstream to balance the hemostatic function of clotting factors and reduce the formation of unnecessary clotting and embolisms. Naturally occurring coagulation inhibitors include the following substances: antithrombin III, protein C, protein S, and antithromboplastin. **Acquired coagulation inhibitors** are antibodies that act on clotting factors and phospholipids by neutralizing their action or completely removing them from circulation. The following circumstances can cause coagulation-inhibiting antibodies to form: treatment of bleeding disorders using pooled or commercial clotting factors, autoimmune diseases, malignancy, or pregnancy.

Symptoms exhibited by patients with coagulation inhibitors include the following:

- Minimal or no response to clotting factor therapy
- Bruising
- Abnormal, excess, or spontaneous bleeding, commonly in the GI tract, genitourinary system, retroperitoneum, muscles, or intracranial space
- Compression of nerves or blood vessels causing decreased circulation of extremities, known as compartment syndrome

In addition, the following laboratory values will be present above the normal reference range in patients with circulating inhibitors:

- Prothrombin time (PT)/international normalized ratio (INR)
- Partial thromboplastin time (PTT)
- Fibrin degradation products
- Monoclonal immunoglobulin antibodies

INHIBITOR ASSAYS

Circulating coagulation inhibitors are indicated in patients who are not receiving heparin therapy and present with prolonged **partial thromboplastin time (PTT)** results. Determination of inhibitors begins with a **thrombin time (TT)** assay to evaluate a patient for heparin therapy or to detect a direct thrombin inhibitor.

Following a negative or normal TT assay result, a patient's plasma will be evaluated in a three-step procedure described below, known as mixing studies:

1. Measure the patient's PTT in normal plasma.
2. Prepare a 1:2 dilution with equal parts patient plasma and normal pooled plasma and measure the PTT.
3. Incubate the 1:2 plasma dilution for 30 minutes at 37 °C, and measure the PTT immediately following incubation.

Mixing study interpretations are evaluated based on the correction of PTT results following each step in the process. Result interpretations are defined by the following:

- **Single- or multiple-factor deficiency**: Normal PTT results obtained in steps 2 and 3
- **Factor V inhibitor or lupus anticoagulant**: No correction of PTT results obtained in steps 2 and 3
- **Slow acting inhibitor or anti-factor VIII**: Correction of step 2 PTT result, but no correction of step 3 PTT result

PLATELET AGGREGATION

Platelet aggregation studies assess the function of platelets throughout the coagulation process and aid in the diagnosis of various bleeding, genetic, and myeloproliferative disorders as well as medication side effects and unexplained excessive bleeding or bruising. **Aggregation studies** use various substances known as agonists that elicit a response from platelets to assess their function during each of the following coagulation mechanisms: adhesion to an injury site, release of granule compounds, formation of a platelet plug, and creation of a surface for activated coagulation protein complexes to bind.

The process of platelet aggregation studies includes the addition of various individual agonists to platelet-rich plasma with a standardized platelet count. Platelet responses induced by each agonist is observed via light transmission aggregometry. The following agonists are used in platelet aggregation studies to induce responses in vitro that are similar to those induced naturally in vivo: collagen, thrombin, adenosine diphosphate, arachidonic acid, epinephrine, and serotonin. Light transmission aggregometry expresses platelet activity by recording changes in light transmission in response to agonists in each phase of aggregation. A primary wave is recorded when the agonist binds to its platelet receptors, and a secondary wave is observed due to platelet activation and granule release.

THROMBOELASTOGRAPHY

Thromboelastography (TEG) is a point-of-care assay used to determine the viscoelastic properties of blood clot formation in whole blood samples. This method monitors the dynamics of the complete coagulation process by reflecting the following properties of a blood clot: the start of clot formation, the maximum stability of a clot, and the gradual resolution of a clot due to fibrinolysis. Semiautomated TEG methods measure the physical properties of a forming clot by placing whole blood in a small sample cup containing a thin wire or pin connected to an electrical transducer. As a clot begins to develop, its elasticity and strength change the rotation of the pin. The rotation produced is converted to electrical signals that are measured to produced graphic and numerical results. Parameters measured by TEG include the reaction time, kinetics, angle, maximum amplitude and time of maximum amplitudes, and the clot lysis time. TEG results aid clinicians in the following instances: detecting coagulopathies and excess heparin effects, evaluating and guiding antithrombotic therapy, determining platelet function, and indicating the necessity of blood

8

product transfusion. This assay is most often performed in physicians' offices, in the operating room of cardiac surgeries or liver transplants, and at the bedside during trauma care.

HEPARIN-INDUCED THROMBOCYTOPENIA STUDIES

Heparin-induced thrombocytopenia (HIT) is a condition in which thrombocytopenia arises in response to anticoagulant therapy and predisposes patients to developing a thrombosis. There are two types of HIT: immune (caused by the development of HIT platelet antibodies) and nonimmune (due to a direct interaction between heparin and platelets). Various laboratory assays may be used in conjunction with one another to assess patients for HIT. Declining **platelet counts** following heparin therapy are an indication of HIT. Platelet counts $> 100 \times 10^{12}$/L during the two days following therapy are indicative of nonimmune HIT, whereas immune HIT presents with their lowest platelet counts ranging between 20 and 150×10^{12}/L five days after onset. **ELISA assays** detect IgG antibodies against **platelet factor 4** in patients experiencing HIT. This assay is used as a screening tool for those suspected of HIT and must be confirmed. The **serotonin release assay** is performed via HPLC and is considered the gold standard method for confirming an HIT diagnosis. This functional assay measures heparin-dependent platelet activation and the quantity of serotonin released by platelets activated by reagent HIT antibodies.

DIRECT THROMBIN INHIBITORS

Direct thrombin inhibitors are medications used for anticoagulation therapy that act directly on the thrombin enzyme. The following medications act on the thrombin molecule in different ways:

- **Lepirudin** binds to the active and substrate binding sites.
- **Argatroban** binds directly to thrombin and blocks the active sites.
- **Fondaparinux** accelerates the binding of antithrombin to activated factor Xa.

The most common laboratory assay for monitoring anticoagulation therapy with these medications is the APTT. The target range for patients receiving lepirudin is an APTT result that is 1.5–2.5 times the baseline APTT results obtained before therapy begins. For example, a patient with a baseline APTT result of 30 seconds would expect to see an APTT result between 45 and 75 seconds for their therapeutic range. Lepirudin therapy can also be monitored with the ecarin chromogenic assay that is based on thrombin inhibition. Argatroban is given to patients with HIT in an effort to avoid the formation of emboli. The therapeutic range for argatroban therapy is an APTT result that is 1.5–3.0 times greater than the patient's baseline APTT. Fondaparinux therapy does not require monitoring. However, if monitoring is requested, assays based on the inhibition of factor Xa are recommended.

Immunology and Serology

General Knowledge

IMMUNOLOGY AND SEROLOGY TERMINOLOGY

Thermostable	Unaffected by heat.
Thermolabile	Easily affected by heat.
Physiologic(al)	Related to body functions.
Inactivation	Destruction of biological activity, such as by heat or other agent.
Complement	A group of blood proteins that go through a cascade of interactions as part of immune response.
Reagin	Complement-fixing antibody, IgE immunoglobulin that attaches to tissue cells in the species it derives from and interacts with antigen to cause release of histamine and other vasoactive amines.
Amboceptor	Old term for hemolysin.
Hemolysin	Antibody that binds to red blood cells and lyses them to release hemoglobin.
Cardiolipin	Phospholipid that increases with some disorders, such as autoimmune and coagulation disorders.
Monoclonal	Referring to a single clone; derived from a single cell.
Polyclonal	Referring to multiple clones; derived from multiple cells.

IMMUNE DESTRUCTION OF RED CELLS BY HEMOLYSIS

Hemolysis occurs when the cell membrane is breached and hemoglobin is released into plasma. **Intravascular hemolysis**, which occurs within blood vessels, may result from inherited diseases (G6PD), acquired disease (DIC, TTP), autoimmune disorders, cardiac valvular prostheses, toxins (drugs, snakebite), parasitic disorders, and incompatible transfusions. RBC fragments or schistocytes are observed on peripheral smear. **Extravascular hemolysis** (most common), which happens outside of the blood vessels, occurs when antibodies attach to RBCs or the RBCs have abnormal morphology and are attacked prematurely and destroyed by phagocytosis in the spleen and liver. Mildly abnormal RBCs may be destroyed in the spleen (which can also sequester RBCs), but the liver has a superior blood supply and is able to more effectively destroy markedly abnormal RBCs. Hemolysis may result from a number of different pathogens, especially gram-positive microorganisms such as staphylococci, streptococci, and enterococci. Microspherocytes are observed on peripheral smear.

CLASSICAL AND ALTERNATIVE PATHWAYS FOR COMPLEMENT ACTIVATION

Complement is a group of serum proteins that become activated in response to a foreign substance in the body, producing inflammation and **chemotaxis**, or movement, of phagocytic cells to the site of infection. The process of coating target cells for the enhancement complement attachment to phagocytic cells is known as **opsonization**. Activation of complement is achieved through different avenues based on the biologic interaction between a foreign substance and the immune system.

The **classical complement pathway** is activated by the formation of an IgG or IgM antigen–antibody immune complex on the surface of foreign material and begins with the esterase inhibitor,

10

C1; the binding protein, **C4**; and a serine protease, **C2**. Complement's **alternative pathway** requires lipopolysaccharides or polysaccharides on that surface of microbes for activation of **C3**.

The classical and alternative pathways converge at the convertase protein, C3, which cleaves into C3a and C3b. **C3a** stimulates inflammation and the release of histamines from complement bound material of the classical pathway. **C3b** binds to microbial cell walls in the alternative pathway, attracting macrophages for the ingestion of the microbe. Following the cleavage of C3, the convertase **C5** is formed, further inducing inflammation and cell lysis with the membrane attach complex.

IMMUNE RESPONSE

The immune system's first response to a foreign antigen is the **primary response**. In the primary immune response, there are no circulating antibodies immediately detectable. IgM antibodies are present between 10 and 14 days after immunogenic antigen stimulation. The body's response to a second exposure to the same antigen is known as the **secondary response**. During the secondary immune response, lymphocytes induce an immediate antibody response and detectable amounts of IgM antibody are rapidly present in serum or plasma, followed by detectable IgG antibodies.

T lymphocytes mature in the thymus from CD34+ progenitor cells and participate in cell-mediated immune responses. T cells differentiate into subpopulations with specific functions that include cytotoxicity and the secretion of cytokines. Making up the majority of lymphocytes circulating in peripheral blood, T cells participate in allograft rejection, graft-versus-host reactions, and delayed hypersensitivity. **B lymphocytes** mature from hematopoietic stem cells in the fetal liver and adult bone marrow and contribute to humoral immunity and the adaptive immune system. B cells differentiate into active plasma cells that form and secrete immunoglobulins, and inactive memory B cells that participate in secondary immune responses.

Macrophages participate in the induction of immune responses through antigen presentation and phagocytosis. Embedded in tissues, macrophages are attracted and adhere to foreign organisms by chemotaxis. Macrophages then engulf the foreign material and destroy it with digestive enzymes found in the cells' granules.

ANTIBODY PRODUCTION

B cells contain antigen receptors (BCRs) and T cells contain antigen receptor (TCR). Immunoglobulins (globular glycoproteins) are antibodies that can bind to antigens as part of activated immune response. Immunoglobulins are found in body fluids and on the surface of B cells. When the B cells are activated by contact with an antigen, the B cells proliferate and begin to differentiate into plasma cells, which produce antibodies:

- IgG—75-80%: Can be transported across the placenta and is the main immunoglobulin produced for secondary immune response and the only one with anti-toxin activity. Present in mucous membranes.
- IgA—15-20%: Primary antibody at mucous membranes where it prevents antigens from entering the immune system rather than destroying them.
- IgM—5-10%. Primarily found in peripheral circulation and is the main immunoglobulin produced for primary response and may be the only antibody produced against some antigens. Present on most mature B cells.
- IgD—0.2%: Found with IgM on many B cells, and its function is not yet clear.
- IgE—Trace. Most is bound to mast cells and basophils and is associated with allergic response.

FACTORS AFFECTING ANTIGEN-ANTIBODY REACTIONS

Factors affecting antigen-antibody reactions include:

Factor	Effect
Temperature	Antigen-antibody reactions are usually more stable at low temperatures, and the strength of bonds tends to increase as the temperature rises.
pH	Equilibrium constant is attained at 6.5-8.4. Extremes alter the antibody molecule.
Incubation time	Duration needed to reach equilibrium varies according to the ionic strength—faster at low strength and slower at high strength. Duration should be at least 20 minutes at low strength.
Ionic strength	Reactions vary in time needed to reach equilibrium depending on the concentration of ions. At low strength, gamma globulins aggregate, resulting in increased complement fraction attachment and RBV aggregation.
Antibody/ antigen excess	Numbers of antigens or antibodies are so high that antigen-antibody crosslinking (agglutination) is reduced because of the excess of either antigens or antibodies.
Enhancement media	Reaction may vary depending on the type of enhancement media utilized.
Blood-banking technology	Rare blood types may cause unexpected reactions.
Dilution/ Concentration	Can alter the number of immunoglobulins by increasing or decreasing dissociation.

HLA SYSTEM

HLA stands for human leukocyte antigen. The human leukocyte antigens are part of the major histocompatibility complex (MHC), a region found on chromosome 6. HLAs are found in all nucleated cells in the body. HLAs are inherited from one's parents and are practically unique to a particular individual. There are four main types of human leukocyte antigens, HLA-A, HLA-B, HLA-C, and HLA-D. Human leukocyte antigens help encode proteins on the surfaces of nucleated cells, and they play an important role in helping the body distinguish its own cells from foreign cells. Therefore, HLAs are very important when it comes to human organ transplant rejection or acceptance. In the laboratory, HLA-A, HLA-B, and HLA-C antigens can be identified using blood serum, however, HLA-D antigens can only be identified by the use of a mixed lymphocyte culture.

Serological Tests for Syphilis

SYPHILIS

Syphilis is a bacterial infection caused by the spirochete *Treponema pallidum* and transmitted through oral, anal, or vaginal sex or needle sharing. The incubation period is 10 to 90 days. There are 3 stages to the disease:

- **Primary** (3-8 weeks): Chancre (painless) in areas of sexual contact, very contagious.
- **Secondary** (1-2 years): General flu-like symptoms (sore throat, fever, headaches) and red papular rash on trunk, flexor surfaces, palms, and soles, hair loss, and lymphadenopathy occur about 3-6 weeks after end of primary phase and eventually resolves.

- **Tertiary/Late** (latent >2 years): Affects about 30% and includes CNS (psychoses, confusion, ataxia, aphasia) and cardiovascular symptoms 3-20 years after initial infection. Gummas (granulomatous lesions) may be widespread. Complications include dementia, meningitis, neuropathy, and thoracic aneurysm. Noncontagious after 4 years.

Women who are infected may transmit the disease to a fetus, resulting in **congenital syphilis**. The infant may be born with no obvious symptoms at birth or may be born with physical changes associated with advanced syphilis.

MICROHEMAGGLUTINATION TEST FOR *TREPONEMA PALLIDUM* (MHA-TP)

The microhemagglutination test for *Treponema pallidum* (MHA-TP), a gram-negative spirochete, is a nontreponemal antibody tests that assesses serum for antibodies to syphilis although this particular test has been generally replaced by other tests that are more specific, such as fluorescent treponemal antibody absorption (FTA-ABS), immunoassays, and molecular testing. MHA-TP can be used to confirm a positive diagnosis of syphilis on other tests. MHA-TP is able to detect antibodies to *T. pallidum* and is used for all stages of syphilis except during the first month of infection. One of the problems with MHA-TP is that false positives may occur in the presence of other infections, so it is not specific to syphilis: mononucleosis, Lyme disease, malaria, relapsing fever, leptospirosis, and leprosy. Patients with systemic lupus erythematosus may also have a false-positive on the test.

Analytical Procedures

FEBRILE AGGLUTINATION TESTS

Febrile agglutinins are antibodies that are active at normal body temperature and can cause their antigens (such as RBCs, proteins) to clump when exposed to each other, resulting in a fever. Febrile agglutinins are present in some disorders, such as systemic lupus erythematosus, hemolytic anemia, inflammatory bowel disease, and lymphoma. They may also occur in response to some infections (salmonella, brucellosis, typhoid fever) and when taking some medications (penicillin, methyldopa), so these medications may interfere with test results. To identify an infection, a blood sample is taken when a patient is actively infected (with fever and symptoms) or during convalescence, diluted (20-40 times), and mixed with antigens of a specific infectious microorganism. This sample is then examined to determine if an antigen-antibody reaction has occurred. Increased IgM usually indicates a new infection and increased IgG indicates a chronic infection or history of infection.

C-REACTIVE PROTEIN AGGLUTINATION SLIDE TESTS

C-reactive protein (CRP) agglutination slide tests can be used to screen patients for CRP (qualitative test) or to determine the titer (quantitative test). A number of different test kits are available, so procedures may vary.

Qualitative test	Quantitative test
Add latex solution to positive and negative controls and serum (or diluted and undiluted serum), mix, and agitate for 2 minutes to observe for agglutination (clumping) in serum, a reaction indicating the presence of C-reactive protein.	Mix serum samples to different dilutions in saline and conduct test similar to qualitative method to determine the highest dilution that shows agglutination (positive reaction).

ANTISTREPTOLYSIN SCREEN AND TITER

Antistreptolysin O screen and titer (ASO) identifies the presence of streptolysin O antibodies, which form in response to the streptolysin O enzyme (antigen) secreted by group A β-hemolytic streptococci. The antibodies are present within one week and peak at 2-3 weeks after onset of streptococcal infection. Increased titer is present with strep-associated rheumatic fever, scarlet fever, endocarditis, and glomerulonephritis.

RHEUMATOID ARTHRITIS (RA) TESTS

Rheumatoid factor (RF)	Normal value 0-20 IU/mL
	Assesses for macroglobulin type antibody that is present in connective tissue disease. Non-specific for RA
Anti-citrullinated protein antibody (ACPA):	Normal values: Negative: <20 Weakly positive: 20-39 Moderately positive: 40-59 Strongly positive: >60
	Assesses for autoantibodies against citrullinated proteins, to which those with RA react.
Erythrocyte sedimentation rate (ESR):	Normal values: Age <50: 0-15 mm/h males and 0-25 mm/h females Age >50: 0-20 mm/h males and 0-30 mm/h females
	Inflammation causes increased globulins or fibrinogens, and these cause RBCs to clump and fall to the bottom of a vertical test tube. ESR is nonspecific for RA, but increased ESR may indicate increased inflammation.
C-reactive protein (CRP):	Normal value <1 mg/dL
	Assesses for abnormal glycoproteins, which are produced by the liver when inflammation is present. CRP is non-specific for RA.

SYSTEMATIC LUPUS ERYTHEMATOSUS (SLE OR LE) TESTS

Systemic lupus erythematosus (SLE) is a chronic connective tissue disorder believed triggered by an antibody-antigen immune response to an environmental agent, resulting in widespread damage of vessels and organs, primarily in females. SLE ranges from mild to widely disseminated, and may include arthralgia, "butterfly" rash, arthritis, anemia, leukopenia, visceral lesions, CNS involvement (seizures, headaches, psychosis), fever, and lymphadenopathy. There is no single specific test for SLE, but rather diagnosis is based on the results of a number of imaging studies (x-rays, ECG) and laboratory studies:

- Complete blood cell count (CDC): May show anemia with erythrocytopenia and/or leukopenia.
- Erythrocyte sedimentation rate (ESR): Rate increases with SLE.
- Renal and hepatic function tests: Abnormalities may indicate lesions in the kidneys or liver.
- Urinalysis: Protein may be in the urine with renal lesions.

- Antinuclear antibody test: Presence of antibodies indicates an immune response. While results are not specific to ANA, this test is used primarily as part of SLE diagnosis.
- Renal biopsy: To determine type and degree of kidney involvement.

ANTINUCLEAR ANTIBODY (ANA) TESTS

ANA is used to diagnose autoimmune disorders, primarily SLE, Sjögren syndrome, scleroderma, and rheumatic diseases, which involve multiple body systems. Diagnosis depends on the ANA pattern exhibited and associated antibodies. Laboratories vary in reference ranges. Antinuclear antibodies are autoimmune antibodies that mistakenly target native tissue and cells as foreign. ANA is often done in conjunction with other autoantibody tests, such as anti-DNA and anti-nucleolar.

Results	Testing
Positive or negative: ANA results vary depending on the specific test used and the lab.	Collect serum (3 mL) in red-capped tube for indirect fluorescent antibody (IFA) or immunoassay. Immunoassay is less sensitive that IFA, so initial screening may be done by immunoassay with confirmation testing by IFA.

ANTIGEN DETECTION

Antigen detection for specific organisms is frequently done as part of diagnostic studies. Various tests can be used. Enzyme immunoassays (EIA/ELISA) use various techniques, depending on the target antigen and microorganism. Techniques include binding an antibody (specific to the antigen under study) to a micro-dilution tray and adding the antigen, incubating, and washing it. Then, a second enzyme-labeled antibody is utilized to detect the antigen through a color change. With use of the immunochromatographic membrane, an antigen is absorbed through a nitrocellulose membrane and the color change occurs on the membrane when reagents are added. Latex agglutination tests, in which the antigen is affixed to latex beads, are used to identify carbohydrate antigens that occur on encapsulated organisms. With the Western blot test, antigens are put on a nitrocellulose strip and incubated with the antibody specimen and treated with an enzyme-labeled antibody and color change observed. Western blot is used frequently to confirm diagnosis of HIV.

PREGNANCY TESTS

Human chorionic gonadotropin (hCG) (quantitative)	Negative: <5 mIU/mL	Measures the amount of hCG in the blood. Obtain 1 mL sample in red or tiger-capped tube or 1 mL in heparinized green-capped tube for immunoassay.
	2 weeks: 5-100 mIU/mL	
	4 weeks: 10,000-80,000 mIU/mL	
	5-12 weeks: 90,000-500,000 mIU/mL	
	13-24 weeks: 5000-80,000 mIU/mL	
	26-28 weeks: 3000-15,000 mIU/mL	
hCG (qualitative)	Negative if absent	Measures only presence or absence of hCG and cannot determine weeks of gestation.
	Positive if present	Obtain 1 mL sample in red or tiger-capped tube or 1 mL in heparinized green-capped tube.
hCG urine (home-pregnancy test)	Positive or negative	A test strip of some type is used and color change noted.

Special Procedures

VIRAL/RETROVIRAL LABORATORY TESTS

Cytomegalovirus	Negative: ≤0.9 index	Obtain 1 mL sample in red-capped tube for enzyme immunoassay for antibody detection.
	Indeterminate: 0.91-1.09	
	Positive: ≥1.1 index	
Retrovirus	Negative: 0 present	Obtain 1 mL sample in red or tiger-capped tube for enzyme immunoassay for antibody detection. Tests may include ELISA, nucleic acid testing, PCR, western blot.
Epstein-Barr	Negative: <17 u/mL	Obtain 1 mL sample in gold-capped serum separator tube for chemiluminescent immunoassay.
	Indeterminate: 18.0-21.9 u/mL	
	Positive: >22 u/mL	
Rubella	Negative: ≤0.9 index	Obtain 1 mL sample in red-capped tube for chemiluminescent immunoassay.
	Indeterminate: 0.91-1.09	
	Positive: ≥1.1 index	

ANTI-HUMAN IMMUNODEFICIENCY VIRUS (HIV) TESTS

These tests screen for the presence of antibodies and/or antigens to HIV. The antigen is present before antibodies, so tests that include antigen assessment can give earlier results.

Rapid HIV test	Negative or positive	Most test only for antibodies, but newer tests may test for antigens as well. Tests can be done on blood, plasma, or oral fluid, but the rapid test is most often done with an oral swab with results (usually color change) available within seconds to minutes, depending on the test. These tests are less accurate than other tests, so findings must be confirmed.
HIV-1/HIV-2 test (serum)	Negative or positive	Screens for HIV antigen (p24) and HIV-1 and HIV-2 antibodies. Obtain 1 mL sample in red-capped tube for enzyme immunoassay. Confirmatory tests required.
IFA/Western blot	Negative or positive	Done for confirmatory testing when initial screening tests are positive or with individuals at high risk with negative screening tests.

Immunohematology

General Knowledge

IMMUNOHEMATOLOGY TERMINOLOGY

Antihuman globulin (Coombs)	Animal (commonly rabbit) serum immunized with human globulin that has been purified to prepare antibodies against immunoglobulin G (IgG) and complement.
Direct antihuman globulin test	RBCs washed to remove serum and unbound antibodies and the antihuman globulin added. Agglutination occurs with presence of antibody. Test used to detect sensitized RBCs in erythroblastosis fetalis and autoimmune hemolytic anemia.
Indirect antihuman globulin test	Serum incubated with donor RBCs, cells washed, and antiglobulin added. If cells absorb antibody, agglutination occurs: Used for blood typing and adverse transfusion reactions.
Compatibility testing	Testing carried out between the patient's blood specimen and the donor's blood specimen to ensure the blood types are compatible. Includes blood typing of patient and donor, repeat donor testing, forward, reverse, and weak D (Du) cross match testing and further testing as indicated for discrepancies.
Auto control/ Autoimmunity	Condition in which a humoral or cell-mediated response to components of body tissue (autoantigens) results in hypersensitivity reactions or autoimmune disease in which antibodies attack the body'
Immunogen	Any substance that produces an immune response
Antigen	Any substance that reacts with substances in the immune system; antigens do not always produce an immune response
Hapten	A molecule with a low molecular weight, which combines with another molecule to produce an antibody response
Adjuvant	A substance that magnifies immune responses
Antibody	A protein that fixes itself to an antigen; also known as immunoglobulins, and divided into five classes: IgA, IgD, IgE, IgG, and IgM
Polyclonal hypergammaglobulinemia	A broad spike in the gamma region of the protein electrophoresis performed on a serum; indicates elevated levels of specific antibodies; the result of infectious disease, liver disease, or inflammation
Monoclonal hypergammaglobulinemia	A narrow peak in the gamma region of a protein electrophoresis performed on a serum; due to malignant transformation of a B lymphocyte clone; the results of multiple myeloma, immunoglobulin heavy chain diseases, or Waldenström's macroglobulinemia

IMMUNOGLOBULINS

Immunoglobulins are antibodies produced by B lymphocytes in response to exposure of foreign material in the body. These immunogenic gamma globulin (Ig) serum antibodies are composed of protein and carbohydrates. All glycoprotein antibody classes share the same basic monomer

17

structure consisting of four polypeptide chains in a Y shape. Pairs of identical heavy and light chains are connected to each other at a hinged region by disulfide bonds to form polypeptide chains. Although only two types of light chains, kappa (κ) and lambda (λ), are common to all immunoglobulin classes, there are a variety of heavy chain chemical structures that differentiate Ig classes from one another. Immunoglobulins contain three constant regions on each heavy chain and one on each light chain that remain the same in every antibody. They also contain one variable region located at the terminal end of each heavy and light chain, with differing amino acid compositions relative to each class of antibody. Immunoglobulins are classified by their molecular weight, structure, and biological activity into the following five classes: IgA, IgD, IgE, IgG, and IgM.

PHYSICAL AND BIOLOGICAL PROPERTIES OF IMMUNOGLOBULINS

IgA molecules are between 160,000 and 500,000 daltons in size, contain alpha (α) heavy chains, and comprise 13% of total circulating antibodies. The two subclasses of IgA molecules are IgA1 and IgA2. **IgA1** is primarily found in serum and is a monomer structure, whereas **IgA2** is structured as a dimer that is most often a secretory immunoglobulin present in tears, saliva, and nasal mucosa. The primary function of IgA molecules is to defend against local infections at mucosal surfaces.

IgD molecules are 180,000 daltons in size, contain delta (δ) heavy chains, and make up 1% of circulating antibodies. IgD molecules are monomers that are present on the surface of B cell lymphocytes that signal the cells to begin activation.

IgE molecules are monomers that are 196,000 daltons in size and contain epsilon (ε) heavy chains. These antibodies circulate in serum in trace amounts and act to release histamines from mast cells in response to an allergy.

IgG molecules are 150,000 daltons in size, contain gamma (γ) heavy chains, and make up 80% of the concentration of total circulating antibodies in serum. IgG antibodies are the only class that is able to cross the placenta from mother to fetus. Four subclasses of IgG antibodies exist, each with a functional difference due to their difference in location and number of disulfide bonds at the constant region of their heavy chains: IgG1, IgG2. IgG3, and IgG4. The variation in IgG subclasses allows for a variety of avenues for antigen binding, immune complex formations, complement activation, and triggering effector cells.

IgM molecules are the largest immunoglobulin at 900,000 daltons in size, contain mu (μ) heavy chains, and have a pentamer structure. IgM accounts for 6% of circulating antibodies in serum and are the best immunoglobulin for fixing with complement due to their multiple binding sites. Participating in the early phases of immune responses, an increased concentration of IgM antibodies indicates a current or acute infection in the body.

GRADES OF AGGLUTINATION REACTIONS

Red blood cells can manifest six grades of agglutination reaction:

0	Lowest grade; no agglutinative red blood cells are present
+w	Red blood cell button divides into almost invisible or invisible clumps
1 +	Red blood cell button divides into a number of small and medium-sized clumps
2 +	Red blood cell button divides into numerous medium-sized clumps
3 +	Red blood cell button divides into large clumps
4 +	Red blood cell button does not break into clumps; free red blood cells cannot be seen in the background

AUTOIMMUNE DISEASE

Any condition in which a person creates antibodies for their own antigens is an autoimmune disease. There are a couple of different theories that seek to explain autoimmune disease. The **immunologic deficiency theory** asserts that all of the antibodies produced by B lymphocytes are suppressed by T lymphocytes, and so antibodies are produced any time there is a decrease in T lymphocyte activity. The **forbidden-clone theory** asserts that occasionally lymphocytes erroneously fail to destroy autoantigens during fetal development. The theory of sequestered antigens asserts that some antigens can remain invisible to the immune system until tissue is damaged.

SENSITIZATION IN RELATION TO ANTIGEN-ANTIBODY REACTIONS

In many in vitro antigen-antibody reactions, the first stage is sensitization, the point at which the antibody has attached to the antigen but has not yet produced any agglutination or hemolysis. The optimal pH for sensitization is 7. The degree of sensitization will depend on incubation time, defined as the amount of time in which the antibody has to attach to the antigens. Also, antibodies will react most strongly at a temperature of 37°C. Finally, sensitization will be increased in proportion to the ratio of serum to cells; more serum means more available antibodies.

HEMOLYTIC DISEASE OF THE FETUS AND NEWBORN (HDFN)

Hemolytic disease of the fetus and newborn (**HDFN**) occurs when a baby's RBCs are positive for an antigen that a mother's RBCs are negative for. Most often, HDFN develops due to ABO or Rh incompatibilities, but it can also occur with potentially any RBC-group incompatibility (anti-c, anti-K, anti-E are common). If the baby's blood enters the mother's circulation during pregnancy or childbirth, the mother's immune system will recognize the foreign antigen and subsequently produce IgG antibodies against it. After sensitization of the mother's RBCs occurs, the IgG antibody can cross the placenta and enter the fetus' circulation. Antibodies react with antigens on the baby's RBCs, coat them, and destroy the RBCs, causing anemia and hyperbilirubinemia.

Ultrasound, including color Doppler, and amniocentesis tests for bilirubin and fetal maturity can detect HDFN and its severity in utero. HDFN can also be detected after birth with samples from the mother and/or baby. Tests performed on samples from the mother can include the rosette test or detection of fetal hemoglobin (HbF) via acid elution, chromatography, or flow cytometry.

Samples from the baby may be tested with the following methods: cord blood ABO/Rh, DAT, hemoglobin, peripheral smear, reticulocyte count, and bilirubin levels.

TREATMENT AND PREVENTION FOR HDFN

Treating HDFN can be done in the antepartum or postpartum period depending on the severity of the disease. In mild cases, neonates can be treated with **phototherapy** to clear excess bilirubin from their system. More severe cases may be treated with RBC **exchange transfusions**, with a significant portion of the newborn's blood (most commonly O negative) being transfused with donor RBCs compatible for the mother's blood. **Intrauterine or umbilical vein transfusions** are also an option when delivering the baby is too great of a risk. This will correct severe HDFN and aid in the delivery of a healthy baby.

Prevention of HDFN begins with maternal screening early in pregnancy to establish ABO/Rh type and the presence of antibodies present in her blood. Rh-negative women will be administered **Rh immunoglobulin** at 28 weeks antepartum and within 72 hours after giving birth. Rh immunoglobulin allows for passive immunization of the mother's RBC antibodies and keeps them from attacking incompatible fetal RBCs. Women positive for antibodies due to previous pregnancy

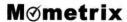

or transfusions will have a titer of that antibody monitored throughout pregnancy to detect an active immune response. If the antibody titer increases, the potential for HDFN arises and must be monitored for its severity.

Blood Typing

GENERAL MOLECULAR STRUCTURE OF AN ANTIBODY

Every antibody has four molecular chains, two light chains and two heavy chains. The light chains contain a variable region in which the antibody bonding site is found. Some antibodies produce agglutination because of their reactions with the antigens on red blood cells. The heavy chains, on the other hand, determine the antibody's immunoglobulin type

ANTIGEN-ANTIBODY INTERACTIONS AND WAYS ANTIGEN-ANTIBODY COMPLEXES ARE HELD TOGETHER

The interactions between antigens and antibodies may result in the formation of a complex. An antigen will bond to the variable region on the light molecular chain of a corresponding antibody. These interactions may be stronger or weaker depending on the compatibility of the antigens and the antibody. In vitro, the reactions between an antigen and an antibody cause agglutination or hemolysis; in vivo, they may result in an immune response. The following forces conspire to hold together antigen-antibody complexes: hydrophobic bonding, hydrogen bonding, electrostatic charge, and Van der Waal's force.

ANTIBODY ENHANCER

An antibody enhancer is the chemical that stimulates the formation of antigen-antibody complexes. For instance, the proteolytic enzymes papain, ficin, and bromelain are frequently used as antibody enhancers, because they increase red blood cell agglutination. Bovine albumin, on the other hand, encourages sensitized red blood cells to form agglutination lattices. Low ionic strength solution, known by the abbreviation LISS, is often used to stimulate the formation of antigen-antibody complexes. Finally, polyethylene glycol additive, or PEG, concentrates antibodies.

H ANTIGEN AS RELATED TO THE A, B, AND O BLOOD TYPES

The H antigen is part of the A and B antigens, functioning as an acceptor molecule for sugars. Blood type A is the H antigen with N-acetylgalactosamine affixed. Blood type B is H antigen with D-galactose affixed. Blood type B is also H antigen with no sugar affixed. Only .01% of the world's population has the h antigen rather than the H antigen, known as the Bombay blood group (phenotype hh). These individuals are universal donors because they lack A, B, and H antigens, but can only be transfused with Bombay blood group blood.

ABO BLOOD SYSTEM

The ABO blood system differentiates based on the amount of A antigens and B antigens on the outside of red blood cells. Individuals who have red blood cells with both A and B antigens on the surface are said to have AB blood. This indicates that such individuals do not have antibodies (IgM) against these antigens in their blood serum. In like fashion, individuals who only have the B antigens on the surface are said to have B blood. Individuals will only have IgM antibodies against the A antigen. Similarly, individuals with type O blood will have red blood cells with neither A nor B antigens on the surface, but blood serum will contain antibodies against both A and B antigens.

RBC ANTIGEN PHENOTYPING AND FREQUENCY OF ANTIGEN DISTRIBUTION

Erythrocyte (RBC) phenotyping is done based on the type of antigen on the cell surface with A, B, AB, and O the 4 primary phenotypes, but there are many other antigens present, and these antigens are not usually tested for with blood typing although it may be necessary for some patients, especially if discrepancies occur with typing or patients have known subtypes or rare blood types (RzR, Jk [a-b], Di [b], Dr [a-]). Antigen distribution (average, USA):

	A	B	AB	O
Rh+	31%	9%	3%	39%
Rh-	6%	2%	1%	9%

Distribution varies according to ethnicity and matching may be easier within the same ethnic group. For example, while 39% of people are O+, this ranges from 37% of Caucasians, 39% Asians, 47% African Americans, to 53% Asians. Indigenous populations in South and Central America are almost 100% type O+.

SCREENING FOR ANTIGEN NEGATIVE BLOOD IN A NORMAL POPULATION AND PROPERLY USING POSITIVE AND NEGATIVE CONTROLS

Antigen-negative blood: While blood typing for the normal population is done for ABO and RH (D) antigens, there are over 300 antigens on red blood cells (RBCs), and patients can develop antibodies to any of these antigens. In most cases the antibody-antigen reaction is so mild it is of no consequence, but severe reactions can occur. These reactions become evident during the thermophase and/or antihuman globulin phases of testing. These patients must receive blood that is antigen-negative for the antigens to which they have antibodies that may result in reaction. For antigens with a fairly high rate of frequency, screening may be done locally, but for more obscure antigens, screening may need to be done in reference laboratories with large numbers of controls available. Negative controls are used for positive presence of antigens, and positive controls for negative presence, and these must carefully match the RBCs or errors will occur.

ANTIGEN DISTRIBUTION AND PROVISION OF ANTIGEN-NEGATIVE BLOOD FOR TRANSFUSION

When a patient has antibodies to specific antigens and must receive antigen-negative blood for transfusion, a problem that most often occurs in patients who undergo more than 15 transfusions and develop antibodies to minor antigens, the number of units that must be tested depends upon the **antigen distribution**. For example, if an antigen is found in about 20% of a population, one can estimate that 20% of units of blood contain that specific antigen (even though the actual percentage may be higher or lower). If a patient must receive 2 units of blood, the formula to estimate the number that must be tested for compatibility is:

$$\frac{[\text{\# of units ordered}]}{[\text{percentage of units containing the antigen}]} = \frac{2}{0.20} = 10 \text{ units}$$

If the patient carries antibodies to more than 1 antigen and must receive blood that is antigen-negative for both types, then the calculations must take both into consideration.

ANTIBODY-ANTIGEN REACTIONS IN THE LABORATORY

Labeled immunoassay: A test in which a label, like enzyme, radionucleotide, fluorochrome, or chemiluminescent molecule, is affixed to an antibody or antigen so that results may be measured

Agglutination reaction: Lab test in which a soluble antigen reacts to a soluble antibody or vice versa; examples may be reactions between different ABO blood types or the hCG agglutination reaction

Precipitation reaction: Laboratory tests in which soluble anti-bodies react with soluble antigens, as for instance the tests radial immunodiffusion, double gel diffusion, immunofixation, immunoelectrophoresis, nephelometry, and turbidimetry

BLOOD TYPING

- **ABO Forward**: Reagent that contains anti-A and anti-B antibodies used to determine presence or absence of A and/or B antigens on surface of erythrocytes.
- **ABO Reverse**: Reagent that contains A1 and B antigen used to test serum for anti-A and/or anti-B antibodies to confirm forward testing. Any discrepancy must be resolved before blood transfusion. For example, the patient may have the A2 subgroup and may require additional testing to identify that subgroup.
- **D (Rh)**: Rh+ individuals carry the D antigen and Rh- do not, but the anti-D antibody is not naturally occurring but occurs as part of the immune response when Rh- blood comes in contact with Rh+ blood, such as may occur during pregnancy when Rh+ fetal cells pass into maternal circulation or from a transfusion. Erythrocytes are tested with a reagent with anti-D antibody.
- **Du (weak D)**: Because some D+ cells have a weak antigen and do not react to anti-D antibodies, further testing for the weak D is carried out with the cells incubated, washed and anti-human globulin added to determine if agglutination (weak D positive) occurs.

BLOOD GROUPING SERA AND REAGENT RBCS

In **forward** or **direct blood typing**, blood grouping sera are mixed with patient RBCs and the presence of absence of a reaction is used to determine the blood type. Reactions that indicate the presence of an antigen are agglutination and hemolysis. **Agglutination** is clumping of RBCs, occurring when antigen in patient cells combines with antibodies in reagent antiserum. This reaction occurs at various strengths and is graded (0 to 4+) depending on its strength. **Hemolysis** occurs when antisera antibodies and patient RBC antigens react with one another's RBCs releasing hemoglobin and producing a clear, cherry-red solution with or without agglutination present.

Reagent RBCs coated in A1- and B-cell antigens and suspended in saline are used to perform **reverse blood type** testing on patient serum. Reactions for reverse type testing are based on the presence or absence of agglutination. No agglutination indicates no serum antibody to the specific reagent antigen, and an agglutinant reaction of varying strengths (0 to 4+) indicates that a serum antibody to the reagent antigen is present.

EXAMPLES OF BLOOD GENOTYPES AND PROBABILITY OF BLOOD TYPES

Mother	Father	Offspring Genotypes	Blood Type Probability
AB	AO	AA, AO AB BO	A: 50% AB: 25% B: 25%
BO	BO	BB, BO OO	B: 75% O: 25%

22

Mother	Father	Offspring Genotypes	Blood Type Probability
OO	AO	AO OO	A: 50% O: 50%
AO	BO	AB AO BO OO	AB: 25% A: 25% B: 25% O: 25%

Immune Response

ANTIGEN–ANTIBODY INTERACTIONS

In an immunocompetent host, organisms and other sources with antigenic properties will induce a response from antibodies. Foreign antigens are recognized by lymphocytes and stimulate the plasma cell production of antibodies that are specific to the epitopes, or antigenic determinants of a foreign antigen. After antibody production, the variable portion of its polypeptide chain, known as the paratope, recognizes the antigen-specific epitopes. The antibody paratope is created with a high affinity for its specific antigen's epitope that will cause the antigen and antibody to bind together in a lock-and-key manner. The type of weak, noncovalent bond formed between the antigen and antibody is determined by the site on the antibody where the bond takes place. The following bonds and interactions are typical of antigen–antibody complexes: electrostatic bonds, hydrogen bonds, van der Waals forces, and hydrophobic interactions. The immune complex formed by antigen–antibody interactions is transported to cellular systems, most commonly macrophages, to be destroyed or deactivated.

ANTIGEN–ANTIBODY INTERACTION TESTING

The presence or absence of an antigen–antibody complex can be visually observed due to agglutination and precipitation. Agglutination and precipitation rely on the aggregation of test antigens with the corresponding antibodies present in a sample. If the antibody is present, the test antigen will bind to the antigen-binding fragment site of two antibodies and create a lattice formation resulting in the visible end product. **Precipitation** testing methods use soluble test antigens that will aggregate with an antibody to cause a precipitate to settle out of a solution. **Agglutination** methods are based on the use of particulate antigens forming a bridge between antibodies, resulting in clumping. Agglutination occurs in two stages, sensitization and lattice formation. **Sensitization** represents the physical attachment of antibodies to antigens and is dependent on certain physical conditions such as pH, temperature, and incubation period. It is imperative to know the properties of specific antibodies because each one reacts best at different pH levels, temperatures, and with or without periods of incubation. Once the sensitization phase is complete, cross-links between sensitized antibodies will result in aggregation during the final phase of lattice formation.

Clumping due to precipitation or agglutination indicates the presence of the suspected antibody in patient serum, aiding in the diagnosis or establishment of exposure to a particular antigen-bearing entity. The absence of a precipitant or agglutinin determines the lack of a specific antibody in serum.

Precipitation Testing Methods

Single or **radial immunodiffusion** is used to determine the concentration of antigen present in a serum sample. Antibodies are imbedded in the agar of a plate with circular wells, where patient serum and known standards are added. The plate is incubated, and diffusion occurs, forming rings of precipitate around the wells. The diameter of each ring is measured and compared on a plotted standard curve, where the concentration of antigen present in the sample is able to be determined.

Double immunodiffusion or **ouchterlony** methods are used to determine a relationship between an antigen and an antibody. A known antibody is added to the wells of an agar plate, with patient sera and known standards added to its surrounding wells. The plate is incubated and diffusion occurs, resulting in a visible band of precipitation. The location of precipitant bands from patient wells is compared to standard wells to determine antigen–antibody identification.

Immunoelectrophoresis uses gel diffusion and electrophoresis to determine the heavy and light chains in immunoglobulins. The trough of the agar is filled with known antibody that is diffused across the gel by electrophoresis with patient serum proteins. At the zone of equivalence, a precipitation arc appears, and the size of the arc is determined by the concentration of antigen present.

Immunofixation combines protein electrophoresis and immunoprecipitation to classify monoclonal gammopathies by determining the heavy and light chains involved. Patient serum is added to six positions on the agarose plate that are electrophoresed to separate proteins. Monospecific antisera are added to five of the lanes, leaving the sixth lane as a reference. If antigen is present in patient sera, bands of antigen–antibody complexes precipitate, wash, and stain, to become easily visible and able to compare to reference immunoglobulin bands.

Agglutination Testing Methods

Direct agglutination detects antibodies against cellular antigens. A known antigen in the form of an insoluble particulate is added to the patient sample. If antibodies for the antigen are present, an antigen–antibody complex will form and visual clumping is observed. If the antibody is not present, there will be no agglutination in the test field.

Passive hemagglutination uses a soluble antigen to detect an RBC antibody. A patient samples suspected of containing an RBC antibody is serial diluted, and a suspension of reagent RBCs is added to the sample. Cross-links will form between RBCs and visual agglutination will be observed if the antibody is present in the sample. If no antibody is present, the RBC suspension will fail to agglutinate.

Passive latex agglutination uses latex beads coated in soluble reagent antigen to act as a passive carrier. The latex beads are combined with the patient sample to establish the presence or absence of the specific antibody to the reagent antigen. Visible aggregates of the latex beads will form when the antibody binds to antigens on the surface of the beads. If there is no antibody present in a sample, no binding will occur and the latex beads will not agglutinate.

Types of Immune Response

Innate (first line of defense): Available at birth as a first-line nonspecific defense against foreign pathogens and able to respond rapidly because it is not antigen dependent. The innate immune response includes barriers, such as the skin (epithelial cells), body oils (acidic), mucus (acidic), and stomach acid. In addition to barriers, the innate response includes an inflammatory response with phagocytosis (macrophages, neutrophils, dendritic cells). Natural killer cells kill pathogens. Mast cells stimulate cytokine production. The innate immune response activates the adaptive response.

Activated (second line of defense): Involves the antigen-antibody responses. B lymphocytes stimulate the humoral response (antibody production) and T lymphocytes the cell-mediated response (antigens attacked and lymphokines secreted. Initially develops slowly as antibodies form in response to foreign antigen, but antibodies stay in the system and can be mobilized quickly with subsequent exposure.

ACUTE PHASE REACTION

The acute phase reaction is part of the innate immune response when disturbance, such as infection or trauma, occurs. Phases include:

- Injury causes mononuclear phagocyte activation.
- Pro-inflammatory cytokines (glucocorticoids and nitric acid) released.
- Inflammatory cells activated.
- Hypothalamic-pituitary axis activated, resulting in changes in blood chemistry and fever, loss of appetite, and changes in sleep patterns.
- Vascular permeability and adhesiveness increase. Both prostaglandin synthesis and procoagulant activity increase.
- Liver increases production of acute phase proteins: C-reactive protein (CRP), serum amyloid A, haptoglobin, natural opsonin (MBL), complement proteins (C-3, C-4), ceruloplasmin, ferritin, fibrinogen. These proteins bind to microorganisms, modulate the immune response, binds to erythrocytes, and increases clot formation.
- Liver decreases production of storage and transport proteins (transferrin, albumin, transthyretin). The decrease in albumin and transferrin reduces the amount of iron available for microbial growth.
- Muscle and bone tissue breaks down.
- ESR increases because of increased plasma proteins (fibrinogen, immunoglobulins).

FLUID-PHASE PRECIPITATION REACTION

In a fluid-phase precipitation reaction, the antigen and antibody are soluble and tend toward diffusion. The reaction is accomplished as follows: a soluble antigen in solution is placed on top of a soluble antibody in solution, at which point the antigen and antibody diffuse into one another. A precipitate is formed, directly proportional to the concentrations of the antibody and antigen.

TYPES OF IMMUNOFLUORESCENCE REACTIONS

Direct immunofluorescence: reagent antibody labeled with fluorescent dye reacts to a specific antigen, forming an antigen-antibody complex, and thereby suggesting the existence of a particular antigen

Indirect immunofluorescence: unlabeled antibody reacts with antigens and a sample, forming an antigen-antibody complex; at this point, the antigen-antibody complex reacts with another labeled antibody, forming an antibody-antigen-antibody complex

Biotin-avidin immunofluorescence: a form of indirect immunofluorescence in which a labeled antibody and a labeled fluorochrome react with an antigen

KELL BLOOD GROUP SYSTEM

The Kell blood group system is composed of four antigens that are found in red blood cells (erythrocytes). These four antigens are K (Kell), k (Cellano), Kpa, and Kpb. The particular phenotype known as the knull phenotype (K-k-Kp(a-b-)) has been implicated in chronic granulomatous disease (CGD). In this disease, neutrophils cannot produce hydrogen peroxide to kill

25

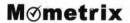

invading bacteria and viruses. The antibodies to the Kell antigens are the IgG antibodies, and IgG antibodies can play a part in hemolytic disease of the newborn, as well as in adverse patient reactions to transfusions.

DUFFY BLOOD GROUP SYSTEM

The Duffy blood group system is a group of antigens (proteins) found on the outsides of erythrocytes (red blood cells). They are distinguished based on their reactions with anti-Fyᵃ serum. Blood can be said to be Duffy positive, meaning that the Duffy antigen is present on the red blood cells. Blood can also be said to be Duffy negative, meaning that there is no Duffy antigen present. There are three common Duffy phenotypes, and they are Fy(a+b+), Fy(a+b-), and Fy(a-b+). Almost all whites are Duffy positive, and almost all blacks of African descent are Duffy negative. Because the Duffy antigen is a receptor for the parasites that can cause malaria, being Duffy negative (not having the Duffy antigen) can help provide resistance against contracting malaria. Furthermore, if a person who is Duffy negative receives blood that is Duffy positive in a blood transfusion, an allergic reaction can occur.

BLOOD GROUP SYSTEMS, ABBREVIATIONS, AND ANTIBODY CLASSES

Group	Abbreviation	Antibody Class
Kell	K	IgG
Kidd	Jk	IgG
Duffy	Fy	IgG
Lutheran	Lu	IgG and IgM
Lewis	Le	IgM
P	P	IgM
MNS	MNS	IgG and IgM
Ii	I	IgM

BLOOD GROUP SYSTEMS ANTIGENS

Kell	K (kell), k (Cellano), Kpa, Kpb, Kpc, Jsa, Jsb, K11 (Cote), Wka, and Ku The most common antigens are K12, K13, K16, K18, K19, K20, and K22
Duffy	Fya, Fyb, Fy3, Fy4, Fy5, and Fy6
Kidd	Jka, Jkb, and Jk3
MNS	M, N, S, s, and U Both of the M and N antigens are associated with glycophorin A; the S, s, and U antigens are associated with glycophorin B

BRUTON'S DISEASE

Bruton's disease is a condition in which there is a deficiency of all 5 major classes of immunoglobulins. This disease is sometimes referred to as agammaglobulinemia. It is a recessive, X-linked disorder that affects only males. A patient with Bruton's disease does not produce B lymphocytes. Patients will have recurrent pneumonia and sinusitis, poor growth, bowel disease, encephalitis, and may die by age 40. Bruton's disease can be detected by amniocentesis. Patients who get IgG injections by age 5 have less morbidity and mortality. In the laboratory, serum levels of IgA, IgD, IgE, and IgM antibodies may not be detected, and IgG antibodies may also be absent or barely detectable. However, the lack of a gamma globulin peak during serum electrophoresis can indicate the existence of Bruton's disease.

Types of Antibodies

Naturally occurring antibodies are those found in the body that were not produced in response to an antigen but through cross-reactivity or exposure to environmental agents with properties similar to antigen, such as dust and bacteria. Naturally occurring antibodies are usually IgM.

Cold agglutinins (cold-reacting) are autoantibodies (primarily IgM) that activate and cause red blood cell agglutination at cold temperatures (0-10 °C). Cold agglutinins may cause severe hemolytic reactions during transfusions. Cold agglutinins are primarily associated with *Mycoplasma pneumoniae* infection, viral infections, and lymphoreticular cancers. Pathogenicity is dependent on the cold agglutinins' ability to bind to RBCs and to activate complement. Normal findings: Agglutination not evident with titers ≤1:16.

Febrile agglutinins (warm-reacting) are autoantibodies (primarily IgG) that activate at normal body temperature. Febrile agglutinins are associated with lymphoma, leukemia, and a number of infectious diseases, include salmonellosis, brucellosis, tularemia, Rocky Mountain spotted fever, and murine typhus. Normal findings: Agglutination not evident at titers ≤1:80.

Distinctive Aspects of Blood Groups

- Resistance to malaria infection: Duffy blood group; phenotype Fy(a-b-) is most resistant
- Hemolytic disease of the newborn: Related to Rh, ABO, Kell, MNS, and Duffy blood group systems
- Infection with Mycoplasma pneumoniae: Related to Ii blood group system
- Chronic granulomatous disease: Related to Kell blood group system, especially phenotype K-k-Kp(a-b-)
- Paroxysmal cold hemoglobinuria: Related to P blood group system, especially the Donath-Landsteiner antibody

Direct Antiglobulin Test (DAT)

The direct antiglobulin test (DAT) detects either IgG antibodies in their blood sample or complement proteins affixed to red blood cells. The test is performed as follows: red blood cells are washed three times with a saline solution, after which antihuman globulin is added. Agglutination at this point indicates the presence of either complement proteins or IgG antibodies. A DAT is often performed in cases of hemolytic disease of the newborn, autoimmune hemolytic anemia, or transfusion reaction.

Indirect Antiglobulin Test

The indirect antiglobulin test (IAT) measures the sensitization of red blood cells in vitro. The test is performed as follows: patient's blood serum is mixed with red blood cells and incubated at body temperature. Once the IgG antibodies in the serum have had a chance to attach to the red blood cells, the mixture is washed and antihuman globulin is added. Any agglutination indicates IgG antibodies. A false negative may occur when the washing is not done properly or when antihuman globulin is not added to the solution. A false positive may occur when red blood cells are agglutinated before being washed.

Antibody Detection and Identification
Antiglobulin Sera

Antisera reagents are a highly purified solution of an antibody used to detect the presence of antigens on human RBCs. Named after their antibody of detection, antisera reagents can be prepared from monoclonal hybridization or through deliberate animal inoculation of antigen, resulting in a purified antibody serum. **Monoclonal hybridization** fuses one clone of human neoplastic antibody-producing cells with splenic lymphocytes from rodents that have been sensitized. Both methods of antisera production allow for standardized and purified antibody concentrations to a specific antigen.

Antisera reagent standards that must be met include the following:

- Antibody specific with proper concentration of antibody to detect antigen
- Meets a certain strength of reaction with corresponding RBCs
- Sterile, clear
- Container with a dropper, labeled with an expiration date
- Stored at 4 °C when not in use
- Manufacturer directions are to be followed; quality assurance procedures must be established and documented.

ENZYMES

Patient RBCs can be pretreated with enzymes to aid in identifying clinically significant antibodies. **Papain, bromelain, ficin,** and **trypsin** are the proteolytic enzymes used in treating the cells by removing the sialic acid layer of the RBC membrane, allowing more antigenic sites to become available for antibody binding. The use of enzymes aids in antibody identification because of their ability to enhance weakly reacting antibodies and one or multiple antibodies if they are present, while diminishing the reaction of other antibodies. Enzyme-treated cells are tested in an antibody panel, and the results are compared to the untreated patient results to identify an antibody or antibodies present.

- The following antibodies are **enhanced** by enzymes: Kidd, Rh, Lewis, I, P_1.
- The following antibodies are **destroyed** by enzymes: M, N, S, s, Duffy.

ENHANCEMENT MEDIA AND LECTINS

Enhancement media are used to promote antibody binding for an increased ability to detect antigen–antibody interactions. Bovine serum **albumin** promotes antigen–antibody binding by dispersing ionic charges on the RBC surface and decreasing the zeta potential. **Low-ionic-strength saline** includes albumin and glycine to decrease the zeta potential near the RBC surface and increase antibody uptake. **Polyethylene glycol** enhances the interaction between RBCs and antibodies by excluding water molecules from the area surrounding the surface of the RBCs. Removing water molecules from the cell surface area allows RBCs to move closer together, concentrating the antibodies and increasing the antibody uptake.

Lectins are proteins derived from the seeds of plants with ABO blood group specificity that act similarly to IgM antibodies. The proteins are used as commercial antisera to distinguish ABO subgroups and aid in the workup of polyagglutination syndromes. Each lectin has a unique characteristic pattern and reaction against RBCs carrying a particular antigen; for example, *Dolichos biflorus* lectin differentiates A_1 RBCs from the A_2 subgroup by positively reacting with only A_1-coated RBCs.

ADSORPTIONS AND ELUTIONS

The method of **adsorption** is used to bind antibodies to RBCs, removing them from plasma, allowing for the analysis and identification of antibodies that may have been masked. This testing method is also a tool for confirming an antigen's presence on RBCs or an antibody's presence in plasma. **Autoadsorption** methods are used to remove autoantibodies from patient plasma through

28

Copyright © Mometrix Media. You have been licensed one copy of this document for personal use only. Any other reproduction or redistribution is strictly prohibited. All rights reserved. This content is provided for test preparation purposes only and does not imply an endorsement by Mometrix of any particular political, scientific, or religious point of view.

the use of the patient's own RBCs. Most commonly, autoadsorption testing is completed to reveal and identify underlying alloantibodies by removing the interference of warm autoantibodies. **Alloadsorption** methods use reagent RBCs with specific antigens on their surface to remove certain alloantibodies from patient plasma, allowing analysis of underlying alloantibodies to be performed.

Elution methods are used to break the antigen–antibody bond on patient RBCs and release the antibody into a solution. The solution is centrifuged, and the supernatant containing free antibodies, deemed the **eluate**, is tested to determine the antibody specificity. ABO antibodies are often established using an elution method in which the sample is frozen, thawed, and heated, whereas alloantibodies and warm autoantibodies are commonly eluted using an acid solution such as acidic glycine. Elutions are used in complex antibody workups, warm autoantibody detection, HDFN, and during the investigation of transfusion reactions.

TITRATIONS AND CELL SEPARATIONS

Titrations determine the concentration of an antibody in patient serum and the strength of an antigen's expression on RBC samples. The patient sample is serial diluted into tubes with the following dilution of serum to saline in each tube: 1, 2, 4, 8, 32, 64, 128, 256, and 512. Two drops of each dilution and one drop of reagent RBCs coated in antibody-specific antigens are combined in clean test tubes labeled with the corresponding dilution. Each test tube is centrifuged and examined macroscopically for agglutination. Antibody concentrations, or **titers,** are determined by the highest dilution of sample that has an observed reaction of 1+ agglutination.

Reticulocyte cell separation is performed on samples from recently transfused patients to distinguish the patient's native RBCs from donor RBCs in circulation. Reticulocytes are immature RBCs released from the bone marrow that are less dense than mature RBCs. This method uses the differing cell densities to differentiate patient and donor cells. Capillary tubes of the patient sample are centrifuged resulting in mature donor cells settling at the bottom of the tube and less dense immature patient cells remaining at the top. Patient reticulocytes separated off can then be tested for RBC antigens originating from the patient without contamination from donor cell antigens.

ELISA AND MOLECULAR TECHNIQUES

Enzyme-linked immunosorbent assay (ELISA) is used in testing donor blood samples for transfusion-transmitted diseases including HIV, hepatitis, and syphilis. ELISA methods rely on the formation of antigen–antibody immune complexes to determine the presence of potentially harmful substances in blood donor samples. The antibody to specific disease-causing antigens is imbedded in the ELISA area, the sample is added, and finally a chromogenic substrate is added to the test area. If the distinct antigen is present, the reagent antibody will bind with it on one side and an enzyme-labeled antibody will bind to the other creating an antibody–antigen–antibody "sandwich." The addition of chromogenic substrate will induce a color development of the immune complex to determine the presence of potentially harmful antigens in a sample.

Molecular techniques are used to more accurately identify RBC antigens in patients that are commonly transfused, in samples with weak or discrepant reactions, and for antigens that don't have a reliable antiserum. The **polymerase chain reaction (PCR)** is a common molecular method that amplifies a specific region of deoxyribonucleic acid (DNA) that contains the nucleotides that encode each individual antigen. DNA analysis of a sample will determine the presence or absence of the RBC antigen being tested for.

THIOL REAGENTS AND IMMUNOFLUORESCENCE

Thiol reagents dissolve the disulfide bonds made between cysteine amino acids of IgM antibodies and Kell antigens. **Dithiothreitol**, **2-mercaptoethanol (2-ME)**, and **ZZAP**, a mixture of papain and dithiothreitol, are the thiol reagents most commonly used. The use of thiol reagents allows for the IgG antibodies to be distinguished from IgM by diminishing the activity of IgM antibodies while leaving IgG antibodies unaffected.

Immunofluorescence testing methods use the binding point of a specific antibody to determine the presence or absence of its corresponding antigen. The binding point, or epitope, of the reagent antibody is labeled with a fluorescent dye that will fluoresce if the specific antigen binds to the antibody, indicating its presence in the patient sample. Immunofluorescence techniques may be used for testing donor blood units for transfusion-related diseases.

SOLID PHASE AND COLUMN AGGLUTINATION TESTING

Solid phase testing determines incompatibilities between plasma antibodies and target RBC antigens. Patient plasma is added to a microwell with a reagent antigen bound to the bottom of the well. Solid phase tests rely on the Fc portion of an antibody in patient plasma attaching to reagent antigens imbedded in the well. Immune complexes formed in a **positive reaction** cause RBCs to diffuse along the bottom of the microwell in a carpet-like appearance. Unbound reagent cells indicate a **negative reaction** by forming an RBC button on the bottom of the well. Solid phase testing can be used with automated systems for blood typing and antibody identification procedures.

Column agglutination, or **gel testing**, uses reagent RBCs and patient plasma added to the top of a viscous gel matrix in individual wells of a gel testing card. The card is incubated and centrifuged, and the reactions in each well are observed and interpreted. Patient samples that do not bind with reagent RBCs will completely settle to the bottom of the gel column for a **negative interpretation**. Agglutination and IgG binding of a **positive antigen–antibody reaction** inhibits RBCs from moving through the matrix, causing them to settle higher in the gel. Patterns of positive and negative antigen–antibody reactions between patient plasma and antigen-coated reagent cells are interpreted to determine blood types, antibody detection and identification, and crossmatch compatibility.

CHLOROQUINE DIPHOSPHATE AND EDTA GLYCINE ACID

Chloroquine diphosphate (CDP) and **EDTA glycine acid (EGA)** are reagents used to dissociate IgG antibodies from the surface of RBCs in samples with a positive direct antiglobulin test (DAT). The purpose of dissociating IgG from the RBC membrane is to be able to accurately phenotype patient RBCs. Whereas CDP is able to release IgG bound to RBCs without destroying the surface of the membrane, EGA reagents cause damage to certain antigens on the RBC surface. The main antigens that EGA destroys are from the Kell blood grouping system, making it impossible to phenotype for Kell antigens from an EGA-treated sample. CDP- and EGA-treated samples are commonly used in elutions and autoadsorptions in patients with warm autoimmune hemolytic anemia and in cases of HDFN.

Compatibility Testing

CROSS MATCHING

Cross matching is a test to determine if a unit of donated blood will be compatible with the blood of the intended recipient. There are two types of cross matching, major and minor. Major cross matching uses red blood cells from the donor's blood and the serum of the recipient to detect ABO compatibility or incompatibility, and to determine if the recipient's blood serum contains an antibody that will act against an antigen on the donor's red blood cells. Minor cross matching uses the red blood cells of the recipient and the blood serum from the donor. Minor cross matching can also detect ABO compatibility or incompatibility. It determines if the donor's plasma contains any antibodies that may act against antigens present on the surfaces of the red blood cells of the recipient. Minor cross matching is not used frequently.

ANTIBODY DETECTION AND CROSSMATCH TESTING

Antibody screen and panel cells are used in testing patient serum to detect and identify the presence of clinically significant antibodies in a patient's blood circulation. Screen and panel cells are commercially produced group O blood cells with specific antigens present on each of the cells. By testing with different enhancement techniques and at a variety of temperatures, positive reactions to these cells aid in the detection and identification of unexpected antibodies in blood recipient samples that may cause transfusion-related reactions if unnoticed.

Crossmatch testing is performed with recipient serum and donor RBCs to determine if the transfusion of donor cells will be compatible with the recipient's blood in vivo. Immediate-spin crossmatches consist of combining patient serum with donor RBCs in a test tube, centrifuging the sample, and grading the reaction on the RBC button that forms in the bottom of the tube. A negative reaction occurs when the RBC button completely breaks apart with slight agitation of the test tube, resulting in a compatible crossmatch. Positive reactions will result in agglutinated RBCs in patient serum, indicating that donor cells are incompatible for transfusion. In instances in which antibodies are present in patient samples, crossmatches are extended to 37 °C and antihuman globulin (AHG) phases to ensure compatibility with donor RBCs.

DONATH-LANDSTEINER (D-L) TEST

The Donath-Landsteiner test indicates whether paroxysmal cold hemoglobinuria is present. When this condition is present, individuals will contain hemoglobin cold temperatures. The roots of this disorder are in the anti-P antibody of the P blood group system. This antibody connects to the surfaces of red blood cells in temperatures below 37°C and at warmer temperatures causes hemolysis. The Donath-Lansteiner test is performed as follows: a test tube of serum and red blood cells is placed at 4°C, while a control to his place at 37°C. The test tube of serum and blood is gradually warmed to 37°C, at which point the tubes are centrifuged. If after centrifuging neither displays an indication of hemolysis, the test is negative. When the tube containing serum and red blood cells shows evidence of hemolysis, but the control tube does not, the test is positive. If both tubes show evidence of hemolysis, the test is rendered invalid.

EXAMPLES DETERMINING IF BLOOD TRANSFUSIONS WOULD BE SUCCESSFUL

Donor	Recipient	Result
A	AB	Successful, no agglutination
AB	A	Unsuccessful, agglutination
O	B	Successful, no agglutination; type O are universal donors
A	O	Unsuccessful, agglutination
O	AB	Successful, no agglutination; type AB are universal recipients

EXAMPLES DETERMINING IF RECIPIENT/DONOR RELATIONSHIPS WOULD BE COMPATIBLE IN A MAJOR CROSS MATCH TEST

Donor	Recipient	Result	Reasoning
O+	A-	Incompatible	Recipient's blood may contain anti-D antibodies; donors blood contains D antigens
A+	AB+	Compatible	Recipient's blood contains neither anti-A nor anti-B antibodies in serum, so donor's blood is acceptable
A-	O-	Incompatible	Recipient's blood contains both anti-A and anti-B antibodies in serum, so A antigens in the blood of donor will agglutinate
AB-	B-	Incompatible	Recipient's blood contains anti-A antibodies in serum, which will agglutinate when mixed with A antigens

ANTIBODY IDENTIFICATION TESTS

Phases of reactivity, phases involved in reacting donor RBCs with recipient's serum for compatibility testing, include:

- **Saline phase**: Donor RBCs are suspended in saline and combined at room temperature with the serum (which contains the recipient's antibodies) to determine if an antigen-antibody reaction (agglutination) occurs. This phase recognizes ABO incompatibility. "Immediate spin" variation includes only centrifugation and examination (no incubation) and takes 5 minutes. Hemolysis during this phase indicates the presence of cold agglutinins. Antibodies that react are usually IgM.
- **Thermophase with protein phase**: RBCs suspended in the antibody serum are incubated for 30 minutes at 37°C with 22% albumin OR with low ionic strength saline (LISS) to enhance agglutination of univalent antibodies, such as Rh (D). LISS requires 15 minutes incubation time. (This phase of testing may be omitted if testing with antihuman globulin is conducted.) Antibodies that react are usually IgM or IgG.
- **Antihuman globulin (Coombs) phase**: Cells are washed and react with AHG reagent, indicating antibody sensitivity. Antibodies that react are usually IgG.

Enhancement media are those used to increase detection of antibodies. Commonly used enhancement media include albumin and low ionic strength solution. (LISS). Polyethylene glycol (PEG) and albumin (22%) may be used together as enhancement media for the direct antihuman globulin (Coombs) test) to aid in differentiating significant from insignificant antibodies as the enhancement media reduces the time needed for incubation as well as promoting agglutination and reducing zeta potential. Both PEG and albumin enhance agglutination, and PEG enhances antibody uptake but can also cause red blood cell aggregation if centrifuged. Enzymes, such as papain and ficin, may also be used to enhance antibody detection.

Rule-out is a procedure used in an antibody screen to determine if antigens are reacting to antibodies. Each cell is assessed as to whether or not it reacted to various antibodies. For example, if the screen shows no reaction between an antigen and the anti-Fy[a] antibody, then this antibody is ruled out.

Rh Immune Globulin

IMPLICATION OF THE RHESUS FACTOR IN RHESUS DISEASE OF THE NEWBORN

In Rhesus disease of the newborn, a pregnant woman who is Rh D negative is pregnant with a baby who is Rh D positive. A tiny quantity of the fetus' Rh D positive blood enters the mother's blood stream. The mother, in turn, creates antibodies against the Rh D antigen in the fetus' blood. These antibodies can then pass back through the placenta to the fetus, and if there are enough antibodies present, they destroy the fetus's red blood cells. The destruction of these red blood cells is called Rhesus disease of the newborn or hemolytic disease of the newborn. A woman's first pregnancy may seem unaffected, but she can be sensitized during it. The disease gets worse with subsequent pregnancies as antibodies increase, unless RhoGAM injections are given preventatively during pregnancy and after delivery.

KLEIHAUER-BETKE TEST

The Kleihauer-Betke test is an acid elution test used to determine the severity or presence of fetal-maternal hemorrhage postpartum. This is accomplished by determining the quantity of fetal red blood cells or hemoglobin present in the mother's blood stream after delivery. This test is performed when a Rh-negative mother has given birth. In this particular test, at a pH of 3.2, a sample of maternal blood is stained with erythrosine B-hematoxylin. Once the stain is applied, the adult hemoglobin (which is soluble in the acid solution) will turn pale. Sometimes the adult hemoglobin is said to become ghost-like. The fetal hemoglobin, on the other end, is not soluble in the acid solution, and remains bright pink. Depending on the amount of fetal hemoglobin present in the maternal blood sample, the appropriate dosage of Rh immune globulin (RhIg) can be administered to the mother to help prevent the formation of Rh antibodies in the mother's blood.

EXAMPLES DETERMINING IF THE MOTHER SHOULD RECEIVE A DOSAGE OF RHIG

Situation	Decision
Rh-positive mother Rh-negative baby	The mother is not a candidate for RhIg because she is Rh-positive.
Rh-negative mother Rh-negative baby	The mother is not a candidate for RhIg because even though she is Rh-negative, she gave birth to a Rh-negative baby.
Rh- and D^u-negative mother Rh-positive baby	The mother is a candidate for RhIg because she is Rh-negative (D^u-negative), and she gave birth to a Rh-positive baby.
Rh- and D^u-negative mother triplets (one is Rh-positive, and two are Rh-negative)	The mother is a candidate for RhIg because she is Rh-negative, and at least one of her triplets is a Rh-positive baby.

Special Tests

ABO DISCREPANCIES

ABO discrepancies occur when forward testing (RBC) does not match reverse testing (serum). Discrepancies can affect either forward and/or reverse testing. Reactions may be too weak or absent, or unexpected reactions may occur. ABO discrepancies may occur because of technical mistakes in carrying out the procedures or because of actual abnormalities of RBCs or serum. Discrepancies between forward and reverse groupings include:

- **Group I**: Reaction is weak or antibodies are absent.
- **Group II**: Antigens are absent instead of antibodies.
- **Group III**: Abnormalities are present in protein or plasma (increased globulin levels) associated with some diseases, such as Hodgkin lymphoma, or from Rouleaux formation (RBC aggregation with RBCs stacked in chains, which occurs with high levels of acute phase proteins (such as fibrinogen), paraproteinemias (amyloidosis, multiple myeloma), and some IV solutions (Dextran and PVP).
- **Group IV**: A variety of problems may occur because of autoantibodies, alloantibodies, and previous transfusions and bone marrow transplantation, including mixed field agglutination in which 2 different populations of cells are noted.

ABO discrepancies that often occur during crossmatching:

- **Rouleaux formation**: Should disperse with serum dilution with normal saline. If still evident, aggregation represents hemagglutination. Note: Dilution may result in inability to detect weak antibodies.
- **Autoagglutination**: Reaction occurs in auto-control tube and may indicate the presence of cold agglutinins, autoantibodies, and alloantibodies. Cold agglutinins (anti-I, H, M, N, P, and Lewis) cause hemagglutination at room temperature, but the reaction ceases at 37 °C (confirming cold agglutinins). Complete antibody screen, and warm plasma and reagent RBCs for 15 minutes at 37 °C and then carry out reverse ABO testing to eliminate interference of autoantibodies and alloantibodies (of foreign RBCs). Autoantibodies, most often produced in response to hemolytic anemias, frequently result in a positive direct antihuman globulin (AHG) test because of the autoantibodies coating the RBCs. The presence of autoantibodies is confirmed by washing the cells with NS, eluting the RBCs, and testing antisera. No agglutination should be noted.

ELUTION AND TYPES OF ELUTION TECHNIQUES

One process that can remove antibodies that are fixed to red blood cells in vivo is called elution. There are three basic kinds of elution:

- Lui freeze-thaw technique: IgM antibodies are removed from the red blood cells of newborn babies
- Digitonin destroys the red blood cells, releasing antibodies
- Intact red blood cell antibody removal (RES): red blood cells are not destroyed, but antibodies are removed using buffers

TESTS TO ELUTE ANTIBODIES FROM RED BLOOD CELLS

When the direct Coombs test is positive, the **heat elution procedure** is indicated. The antigen-antibody bond of cells coated with antigens is disrupted to free the antibodies, which are then collected in saline or 6% albumin solution for testing with reagent cells. Procedures may vary somewhat, depending on laboratory protocol. Heat elution:

1. Wash 1 mL sensitized RBCs 5 times in normal saline to remove free antibodies.
2. Wash again in a volume of saline equal to RBC volume and centrifuge at 1500 rpm for 60 seconds.
3. Test supernatant for free antibodies and repeat last wash procedure until no antibodies are detected. The supernatant of the final wash serves as the negative control.
4. Place volume of saline equal to RBC volume in centrifuge tube and incubate in 56 °C water bath for 10 minutes.
5. Centrifuge (prewarmed cups) at 3400 rpm for 69 seconds.
6. Remove supernatant fluid (should be hemoglobin tinted), which serves as the elute.
7. Test elute for presence of antibodies.

SALIVA TESTING

Saliva and other body fluids may contain a water-soluble blood group substance in about four-fifths of the population. These people are positive secretors. Substances secreted by blood type include: A (A and small amount H), B (B and small amount H), O (H), and AB (A, B, and small amount H). **Saliva testing for secretor status**:

1. Obtain 2-3 mL saliva sample.
2. Place tube in water bath (boiling) for 10 minutes to inactivate enzymes.
3. Cool for short period of time.
4. Place in centrifuge tube and centrifuge for 4 minutes.
5. Prepare 3 tubes and label: A, B, and H.
6. Prepare 2 tubes and label: A, B, and H controls.
7. Place 1 drop of diluted antiserum in each tube (anti-A in A test/control tubes, etc.)
8. Place 1 drop of saliva in each test tube and 1 drop of saline in each control tube and mix.
9. Incubate (room temperature) for 10 minutes.
10. Place 1 drop reagent red cells in each test and control tube (A-1 for A, B for B, and screening cell I or II for H).
11. Incubate (room temperature) for 10 minutes.
12. Centrifuge as needed for saline reaction.
13. Note agglutination. Control tubes should show agglutination and test tubes none if negative secretor status.

Blood Banking and Transfusion Services

General Knowledge

BLOOD BANKING TERMINOLOGY

Packed red blood cells	Red blood cell concentrate with most of the plasma removed. A 350 mL unit usually contains about 200 mL of RBCs and 30 mL of plasma along with 100 mL of a crystalloid solution. A few white blood cells and platelets may remain.
Irradiated red blood cells and platelets	Gamma irradiation of blood products inactivates T lymphocytes, which may cause graft vs host disease. Some RBCs are destroyed but platelet function is retained.
Washed red blood cells	Washing of RBC with 0.9% saline is done in a blood processor or centrifuge to remove plasma, plasma proteins, antibiotics, and other components in order to reduce risk of allergic reaction. However, this procedure results in 10-20% loss of RBCs and shelf-life is reduced to 4 hours if stored at 20-24 °C or 24 hours at 1-6 °C.
Frozen (glycerolized) red blood cells	Glycerol is added to red blood cells through a filter. The glycerolized red blood cells are then spun in a centrifuge and concentrated. The RBCs can then be frozen for up to 10 years.
Deglycerolized red blood cells	Frozen plasma is thawed and "washed" to remove glycerol, which is added when RBCs are frozen but can result in hemolysis if it remains in the RBCs during transfusion.
Leukocyte reduction	T lymphocytes are removed from packed RBCs by centrifugation or filtration to reduce incidence of graft vs host disease in recipient.
Whole blood units	Contains all the blood components. One unit is approximately 450 to 500 mL.
HLA antigens	Human leukocyte antigens are major histocompatibility proteins on the surface of WBCs and are used for tissue typing.
Cryoprecipitate (antihemophilic factor)	Pooled units of plasma containing fibrinogen and other antihemophilic factors used to treat bleeding disorders, such as hemophilia.
Fresh frozen plasma	Plasma is frozen within 6 hours of donation and thawed for administration to control bleeding or to replace plasma. One unit (250 mL) of FFP is derived from 1 unit of whole blood and maintains clotting factors but is free of RBCs, WBCs, and platelets.
Platelet transfusion	Centrifugation separates platelet rich plasma (PRP) from whole blood and the PRP is further centrifuged to remove all but 50-60 mL plasma. Platelet transfusions may be from 1 donor (apheresis) or pooled donors (usually 6). Used for thrombocytopenia, CNS trauma, and patients on ECMO or cardiopulmonary bypass.
Anticoagulants	Products, such as EDTA and heparin, which prevent blood from clotting.
Product pooling	Products, such as plasma, pooled together from multiple screened donors, and cleansed to dissolve viruses.

PHERESIS METHODOLOGIES

Plasmapheresis is a form of hemapheresis in which plasma alone is removed from the blood of the donor. Remaining blood products are returned to the donor, who may undergo this process once every eight weeks.

Plateletpheresis is where only platelets are removed from donor blood. It is performed with an electronic apheresis instrument. Donors may undergo this process once every 48 hours

Leukapheresis is where white blood cells alone are removed from donor blood. It is performed with electronic apheresis instrument. Donors may undergo this process no more than twice a week or 24 times in one year

AUTOLOGOUS DONATION

An autologous donation of blood is one in which an individual donates blood for their own personal use in future transfusions. This system eliminates the possibility of a negative transfusion reaction or the passage of disease. On the other hand, autologous donations are expensive and can be wasteful of blood. There are four kinds of autologous donation: preoperative donation, intraoperative collection, intraoperative hemodilution, and postoperative collection.

EXTRACORPOREAL CIRCULATION AND APHERESIS TECHNIQUES

Extracorporeal circulation is the mechanism used to remove blood from a patient's circulatory system into a mechanical system for a treatment or process and return it back to the patient's circulation. Many therapeutic processes use an extracorporeal circuit to remove waste, administer medication, or oxygenate blood in a patient. **Hemodialysis** and **hemofiltration** are used for kidney failure. The process removes waste products that the kidneys cannot excrete on their own and returns the filtered blood back to the body. **Extracorporeal membrane oxygenation** replicates lung function when the lungs are inundated or are unable to properly oxygenate the body; it treats blood with an anticoagulant and filters it through an oxygenator before returning it to the body via a vein or artery. Allowing for a still heart to be operated on, **cardiopulmonary bypass** mechanisms assume the responsibility of pumping blood throughout the body during open heart surgeries. **Apheresis** techniques use an extracorporeal circuit to remove a specific component of blood and return the remaining components to the circulation. For the treatment of immune system disorders, **plasmapheresis** removes whole blood from circulation, separates the plasma by centrifugation, administers treatment to the plasma, and then returns the remaining components back to the patient. Individual blood components that are donated for transfusion purposes, such as platelets and plasma, are collected via apheresis techniques.

PROSPECTIVE BLOOD DONOR EXAMINATION

The following are the basic examinations and requirements for prospective blood donors:

Temperature	<99.5 °F
Blood pressure	< 180/100
Pulse	50-100 beats per minute
Body weight	≥ 110 pounds
Hematocrit	≥ 38%
Hemoglobin	≥ 12.5 g/dL

Example exclusion periods:

Example	Exclusion period
Malaria	Three years following last infection
Taking aspirin	None for whole blood; 48-72 hours for platelet donation
Viral hepatitis	Permanent deferral
Accutane use	One month after last use
Exposure to the blood of another person	One month following exposure
Taken clotting factors in the past	Permanent deferral
Male prospective donor who has had sex with another male	One year from last sexual contact with a male

EXAMPLES DETERMINING IF DONATING WHOLE BLOOD IS POSSIBLE

Scenario	Decision	Reason
A 33-year-old woman with a hematocrit of 38	Allowed	Hematocrit is above minimum acceptable level of 36
A 48-year-old man who received a blood transfusion 5 months ago	Not allowed	Recent blood transfusion creates possibility of hepatitis transmission; hepatitis B has an incubation period of six months
A 21-year-old woman who received a tattoo 14 months ago	Allowed	Individuals are not allowed to donate blood within 12 months of receiving a tattoo
A 35-year-old man who went on a trip to Nigeria 3 months ago	Not allowed	Individuals who do not take a prophylactic for malaria before visiting Africa may donate within six months of their return; individuals who do take a prophylactic must wait three years from their return

PROCEDURE FOR DRAWING BLOOD

The procedure for **drawing blood from donors** includes:

1. Verify identification.
2. Use standard precautions and standard venipuncture protocols.
3. Draw blood from an antecubital vein, if possible, using a sterile collection unit comprised of a large gauge (16-18) needle connected to a closed system with drainage tube and collection bag.
4. Allow the collection bag to fill with blood by gravity by placing the bag in a mixing unit below the level of the arm. The collection bag contains an anticoagulant to prevent clotting and a preservative, such as CPD. The citrate prevents clots from forming, the phosphate stabilizes the blood pH, and the dextrose provides nutrients to the cells.
5. Check the weight of collection bag to determine when it is filled (usually at about 450 mL).
6. Secure the collection bag and remove the needle.

Note: If for some reason the blood flow stops, a completely new setup and collection unit must be used if further blood is taken from the donor as only 1 needle puncture can be used per unit.

POSSIBLE DONOR ADVERSE REACTIONS

On occasion, an individual will experience an adverse reaction when donating blood. Fainting, nausea, rapid breathing, and dizziness are all common side effects of donation. When these or more severe side effects, like convulsions or heart trouble, occur, the tech should immediately remove the tourniquet and blood collection bag. Cold compresses and smelling salts may be appropriate. In especially severe cases, one should make sure that the individual's airway is open and that his or her pulse rate is normal.

ROUTINE PROCESSING AND TESTING OF DONOR BLOOD

Each unit of **blood** or **blood component** is required to be **labeled** with the following:

- Name of the product (red blood cells [RBCs], whole blood, etc.)
- Type and amount of anticoagulant
- Unit volume
- Storage temperature
- Name and address of the collecting facility and the Food and Drug Administration (FDA) registration or license number
- Expiration date
- Unique donor ID number
- Volunteer, autologous, or paid donor must be denoted
- The following phrases must be present on all blood component labels:
  o Properly identify intended recipient
  o Ŗ only
  o See the circular of information for indications, contraindications, cautions, and methods of infusion.

Routine screening tests performed on donor samples:

- ABO, Rh, antibody screen
- Syphilis
- HIV
- *Cytomegalovirus* (CMV)
- Hepatitis B and C — HBsAg, anti-HCV, anti-HBc
- Human T cell lymphotropic virus 1 and 2 (HTLV-I/II) antibody
- West Nile virus
- *Trypanosoma cruzi* antibodies.

REQUIREMENTS FOR BLOOD BANK OPERATION

Requirements for blood bank operation include:

- Obtaining a blood bank license and renewing annually.
- Being available for inspection upon request.
- Participating in proficiency testing.
- Obtaining qualified director and adequate numbers of other qualified personnel.
- Supervising staff, identifying training needs, and implementing training.
- Having appropriate equipment for all functions.
- Using appropriate infection control practices and disposing contaminated materials appropriately.
- Carrying out a documented review for collection/preparation of all blood components.
- Maintaining a manual that outlines all policies and procedures.
- Maintaining correct and legible records that includes significant steps in procedures, test outcomes, ABO/Rh typing result, and donor records, and carrying out reporting responsibilities.

- Establishing criteria for blood collection, processing, storage, distribution, and testing.
- Labeling in compliance with Code of Federal Regulations.
- Storing blood/blood components appropriately and at correct temperature with temperature monitoring system in place.

TRANSFUSION RECORD DOCUMENTATION AND TRANSFUSION ADMINISTRATION PROTOCOL

Transfusion record documentation must be maintained for at least 5 years and those required for tracing a blood product from donor to disposition maintained for at least 10 years following administration or 5 years after expiration date. Computerized records must be secure and software validated. Records must include all those associated with the donor, recipient, and blood product, including testing (all steps and results), storage, and disposition. The records must be easily accessible and allow for tracing of blood products. Donor records must be maintained and should include information about storage temperatures and visual blood inspections, and preparation of components. Recipient records should include blood type and information regarding antibodies history of transfusions, and adverse transfusion reactions. Records should also be maintained regarding therapeutic phlebotomy, policies and procedures, cytapheresis procedures, antibody identification, quality control, and shipping.

MAINTAINING PROPER RECORDS OF ALL QUALITY CONTROL AND BLOOD BANK PROCEDURES

Proper record keeping and documentation for quality control and blood bank procedures are maintained at 4 different levels:

- **Blood bank polices**: A statement of intent that should include the principles that will be utilized to guide decision-making and procedures and may outline the roles and responsibility of employees as well as financial basis for maintaining the program. An example: Employee practices that ensure blood safety.
- **Blood bank processes**: These should outline the way things happen, including the chain of command and basic methods of dealing with various functions of the blood bank, such as collecting, storing, and distributing blood products.
- **Blood bank procedures**: These are step-by-step explanations of how each blood bank procedure, such as collecting a blood sample or applying a label to a blood product, is carried out, including the equipment and supplies needed.
- **Supporting documentation/Forms**: These should include all forms of documentation that are required and samples to show the correct manner of completing and filling out forms required forms.

MAINTAINING QUALITY OF PATIENT SAMPLES COLLECTED FOR BLOOD BANK TESTING

Preanalytical procedures must be followed to maintain the quality of patient samples collected and stored for blood banking purposes. Expired sample tubes cannot be used, and containers with the appropriate additive for blood bank testing must be collected. Identification of the correct patient is imperative prior to collecting a sample, as is correctly labeling the tube once the sample has been collected. Often, a separate, uniquely identifying wristband will be required for a patient receiving blood products. This wristband's identification number will be placed on all of the patient's blood bank samples and blood products assigned to them for an additional form of identification to ensure that the proper patient is receiving the correct products.

BACTERIAL CONTAMINATION

Occasionally, blood products in storage will suffer a bacterial contamination. The most common type of bacterial contaminant is *Yersinia enterocolitica*. Bacteria of this kind will grow while the product is being stored. Individuals who receive blood products that have been contaminated are likely to manifest symptoms similar to those of an adverse transfusion reaction: fever and chills, e.g. Clots, discoloration, or hemolysis in the blood unit indicates possible contamination.

TRANSPORTATION GUIDELINES

Platelets should be transported at room temperature, and they should not be jostled. Red blood cells must be transported at a temperature between one and 10 °C; it is standard to place red blood cells in a Styrofoam box inside a cardboard box and on ice. Frozen blood components must be shipped on dry ice and wrapped well.

MAINTAINING QUALITY OF BLOOD BANK REAGENTS

The following blood banking reagents are tested with quality control samples on each day of their use to ensure they are functioning properly:

- Blood grouping reagents
- Reverse typing cells
- Antibody screen cells
- AHG reagent.

Decreased activity or complete inactivity of reagents with quality control material indicates deterioration of the reagents that can no longer be used for patient testing. AHG reagent quality is also verified for each sample yielding a negative result. IgG sensitized cells, known as check cells, are added to the negatively reacting sample and will agglutinate in the presence of properly functioning AHG. Check cells do not agglutinate in insufficiently washed samples where residual serum neutralizes the AHG.

Testing procedures implemented by reagent and equipment manufacturers' transfusion service facilities must be followed in a strict manner to ensure the accuracy and quality of blood bank processes. Quality assurance policies require comprehensive training of blood bank technologists as well as routine competency testing to ensure that procedures are properly being followed. Evaluation, validation, and the planning of new processes are also important quality assurance measures.

NEUTRALIZATION AND INHIBITION TESTING

Neutralization and inhibition techniques use soluble antigens to bind with antibodies in a sample in order to allow for other possible antibodies present in a sample to be observed. Antigen-rich reagent serum will bind to certain antibodies present in a sample, effectively inhibiting their ability to bind with reagent red blood cells. By neutralizing these antibodies, other alloantibodies that may have been otherwise "masked" are able to bind with reagent red blood cells and be detected in a patient sample. The following blood group antibodies are commonly neutralized in blood bank testing:

- Lewis
- P1
- Sda
- Chido and Rodgers – C4 complement antibodies

Visible Inspection of Units of Blood/Components

Contamination	Cryoprecipitate	Plasma	Platelets	RBCs
Bacteria	Bubbles, clot, fibrin strains, >opaque	Bubbles, clot, fibrin strains, >opaque	Bubbles, clot, fibrin strains, >opaque, grey appearance	Dk Purple -> black
Bile	Bright yellow -> brown	Bright yellow -> brown	Bright yellow -> brown	----
Color abnormality	Any abnormal color	Any abnormal color	Any abnormal color	Supernatant grey/brown
Hemolysis	Pink -> red	Pink -> red	----	Bright red
Lipids	White appearance, > opaque	White appearance, > opaque	White appearance, >opaque	Lighter red, >opaque
Particulates	Clot, aggregates of cellular material	Clot, fibrin strands, white materials	Clot, fibrin strands, white materials	Clot, white materials
RBC contamination	Lt pink -> red	Lt pink -> red	Lt pink	----

Standards for Blood Components

Standards that blood components must meet to be eligible for transfusion are as follows:

Component	Standard
RBCs	Minimum of 80% hematocrit
Leukocyte-reduced RBCs	$< 5 \times 10^6$ leukocytes per unit
Apheresis RBCs	> 60 g hemoglobin per unit
Apheresis RBCs leukocyte-reduced	> 51 g of hemoglobin per unit
Frozen RBCs	$\geq 80\%$ original RBC concentration glycerol removed before transfusion
FFP	Frozen within 8 hours of collection
Cryo	≥ 80 IU per unit and 150 mg fibrinogen per unit
Single donor and pooled platelets	$\geq 5.5 \times 10^{10}$ platelets per unit and pH ≥ 6.2
Leukocyte-reduced platelets	$\geq 5.5 \times 10^{10}$ platelets per unit $< 8.3 \times 10^5$ leukocytes per unit (single donor) $< 5 \times 10^6$ leukocytes per unit (pooled)
Apheresis leukocyte-reduced platelets	$\geq 3.0 \times 10^{11}$ platelets per unit pH ≥ 6.2 $< 5 \times 10^6$ leukocytes per unit
Apheresis granulocytes	$\geq 1.1 \times 10^{10}$ granulocytes per unit

Temperature Requirements, Additives, and Anticoagulants

Anticoagulants and preservatives added to **RBCs** are typically a combination of citrate and dextrose (citrate phosphate dextrose [**CPD**] or citrate phosphate double dextrose [**CP2D**] solutions). **Citrate** acts as an anticoagulant by binding to calcium in the blood and effectively preventing the coagulation cascade from being activated. **Dextrose** provides an energy source to RBCs for viability. An inorganic phosphate buffer (**A-1**) may also be added to prolong RBC viability by increasing the production of adenosine triphosphate (**ATP**). Blood products containing CPD or CP2D may be stored at 1–6 °C for 21 days, and those containing CPDA-1 may be stored at 1–6 °C for 35 days.

Saline adenine glucose (**SAG**) solutions can be added to RBCs to extend the primary anticoagulant storage (**AS**) stability to 42 days at 1–6 °C. Common SAG uses include:

- AS-1 (SAG plus mannitol) with CPD
- AS-3 (SAG plus sodium phosphate, sodium citrate, and citric acid) with CP2D
- AS-5 (ADSOL).

Blood components are available for transfusion until 11:59 pm (2359) on the date of expiration posted on the unit's label. After expiration, components that are not eligible for rejuvenation must be removed from stock and disposed of into biohazard waste bins.

TRANSPORTING BLOOD COMPONENTS AND VISUAL PROPERTIES OF STORED PRODUCTS

RBCs: 1–6 °C — insulated cooler with cold packs to sustain optimal temperature; cannot have direct contact with cool pack; towels or bubble wrap may be used as a barrier between them.

Platelets 20–24 °C (room temperature) — container insulted from exposure to external temperatures.

Frozen components (fresh frozen plasma [FFP] or cryoprecipitated antihemophilic factor [AHF], more commonly known as cryoprecipitate, or cryo): must be kept frozen using an insulated cooler with dry ice.

During storage, it is imperative that all blood products remain in a closed system to avoid loss of quality and to avoid potential bacterial contamination. Storage at proper temperatures will also aid in reducing contamination risks. Upon visual inspection, RBCs should be a deep-red color, with no cloudiness or clots observed. Platelets, FFP, and cryo should not have any clots or particulate matter observed during the storage process.

PREWARMED TECHNIQUE FOR AVOIDING COLD ANTIBODIES

One of the ways that lab technicians try to avoid cold antibodies is by using what is known as the prewarmed technique. This technique is performed as follows: a drop of panel cells and auto control cells is put into a test tube, which is then warmed for 10 minutes at 37 °C. Simultaneously, a tube of serum from the patient is warmed for 10 minutes at 37 °C. The serum is then added to the warmed panel cells, and the mixture continues to incubate for 30 minutes. At this point, it is washed three times with saline that has been heated to 37 °C. Finally, antihuman globulin is added and the reactions of the materials can be interpreted.

BLOOD COMPONENTS
PACKED RED BLOOD CELLS (PRBCS)

Packed red blood cells (**PRBCs**) are prepared by collecting whole blood and separating the RBCs from the plasma by sedimentation or centrifugation. PRBCs are kept at 1–6 °C until issued for transfusion and cannot be returned to the lab if the seal is disturbed or if the unit temperature exceeds 10 °C. This product achieves the same oxygen-carrying capacity as transfusing whole blood, with less volume of product.

- **Storage/Stability:** 1–6 °C for 21 days with CPD or CP2d, 35 days with CPDA-1
- **Indications:** Low O_2-carrying capacity — anemias, ongoing or massive bleed
- **Expected outcome:** One unit of PRBCs will raise hemoglobin by 1 g or hematocrit by 3%

CRYOPRECIPITATED ANTIHEMOPHILIC FACTOR (AHF)

Cryoprecipitated antihemophilic factor (AHF), more commonly known as cryoprecipitate, or **cryo**, is a cold-insoluble portion of plasma formed when FFP is brought to 1–6 °C, separated from the thawed FFP, and refrozen within 1 hour. Units of cryo must contain ≥150 mg of fibrinogen and ≥80 IU/bag of factor VIII. Clotting factors also found in cryo include von Willebrand factor (vWF), ristocetin cofactor activity, fibronectin, and factor XIII.

- **Storage/Stability**: 1 year after collection at –18 °C, 6 hours at room temperature after being thawed
- **Indications:** Fibrinogen loss due to disseminated intravascular coagulation (DIC) or massive bleeding, dysfibrinogenemia with bleeding
- **Expected outcome**: Clotting in efforts to achieve hemostasis

PLASMA

Plasma separated from cells through centrifugation and frozen within 8 hours of collection is known as fresh frozen plasma (**FFP**). FFP is used to introduce clotting factors to the body when it is deficient. This product must be ABO compatible to the recipient to avoid transfusion reactions to residual RBC antibodies.

- **Storage/Stability**: 1 year after collection at –18 °C, 7 years at ≤–18 °C, 24 hours at 1–6 °C once thawed at 30–37 °C
- **Indications:** Coagulation deficiencies, factor XI deficiencies, congenital deficiencies, warfarin toxicity, massive transfusions
- **Expected outcome**: Clotting in efforts to achieve hemostasis

PLATELETS

Platelets can be collected via whole blood samples or apheresis. Whole blood-derived platelets are collected by a low-speed spin to separate and remove RBCs, followed by a second centrifugation at more rotations per minute to separate platelets and white cells. Plasma forms a supernatant, which is separated, and the remaining elements (platelets, white blood cells [WBCs], and some plasma) are kept for platelet transfusion. Apheresis platelets are separated at collection with an instrument that separates the blood components and returns the remainder to the donor.

- **Storage/Stability**: 5 days at room temperature (20–24 °C) with constant, gentle agitation
- **Indications:** Severe thrombocytopenia or platelet dysfunction, prophylactic use for low platelet count and moderate/high risk of bleeding, massive transfusions resulting in thrombocytopenia
- **Expected outcome** (the average adult):
  o One unit of platelets increases the platelet count by 5,000–10,000/µL
  o One unit of apheresis platelets increases the platelet count by 20,000–60,000/µL

LEUKOCYTE-REDUCED COMPONENTS

Leukocyte-reduced components are prepared by filtration and require a $< 5 \times 10^6$ white blood cell (**WBC**) concentration per unit of product. The purpose for transfusing leukocyte-reduced products is to prevent **human leukocyte antigen (HLA)** alloimmunization, CMV transmission, and febrile nonhemolytic reactions in recipients. Common factors that increase the probability of such reactions include the presence of cytokines released from WBCs, prior alloimmunization to HLA, or other leukocyte antigens.

- **Storage/Stability**: Consistent with recommended storage conditions for each individual product (RBCs, platelets, etc.)
- **Indications**: Recipient with repeated febrile nonhemolytic reactions to blood products
- **Expected outcome**: Transfusion of blood products without adverse reactions

APHERESIS PRODUCTS AND FRACTIONATION PRODUCTS

Apheresis products are collected with a process that separates out a specific component and returns the remaining blood components back to the donor's body. The advantage of collecting products with this method is there are fewer inadvertent WBCs present in donations, reducing the risk of adverse recipient reaction to WBC antigens during transfusion.

Fractionation of blood products occurs across multiple steps. Whole blood is slowly spun to separate RBCs from platelet-rich plasma. From this plasma, one unit of donor platelets and one unit of FFP can be collected. FFP can be further separated into individual clotting factor concentrates, or cryo, by flash freezing and collecting the plasma protein precipitates. Fractionating blood products allows for more direct transfusions, focused on a specific product, effectively introducing less volume to a recipient's system and limiting unnecessary transfusions.

WHOLE BLOOD, WASHED RBCS, AND FROZEN/DEGLYCEROLIZED RBCS

Units of **whole blood** are not typically transfused due to the availability of various individual blood components. Transfusions of whole blood are most often used in cases of severe shock and hypovolemia with ≥25% loss of blood volume. RBCs will increase O_2 levels, and plasma will replace lost volume in recipients.

Washed RBCs are prepared by removing plasma from the product with successive saline washes. Removing residual plasma from RBCs will remove complement and diminish the presence of IgA on the cells. Washed RBCs are transfused in patients with anti-IgA to reduce the risk of anaphylactic shock from IgA in plasma. Neonatal transfusions also use washed RBCs from maternal blood to remove anti-HPA-1a for safe transfusion.

Frozen/deglycerolized RBCs are treated with a 40% glycerol cryoprotective agent that allows RBCs to be stored at extremely low (≤65 °C) temperatures for up to 10 years. Cells must be thawed at 37 °C, and the glycerol agent must be removed prior to transfusion. This preparation is typically performed on autologous donations or rare units, in which there is a lack of high-incidence antigens.

REJUVENATED RBCS AND IRRADIATED COMPONENTS

Autologous or rare RBC units may be **rejuvenated** to extend their date of expiration. A solution is added to a unit of PRBCs to restore metabolites that have been depleted over time, such as 2,3 DPG and ATP. Cells must be washed prior to transfusion to remove inosine, which may be toxic. Rejuvenation may be done at any point in a unit's shelf life and up to 3 days past its expiration to extend the RBC unit's shelf life an additional 24 hours when stored at 1–6 °C.

Blood components are **irradiated** to inactivate donor T lymphocytes and prevent graft-versus-host disease (GVHD). If not inactivated, donor T lymphocytes may recognize recipient cells as foreign and destroy them. Recipients at risk of GVHD include those receiving blood components from a family member, a fetus in utero, and patients who are immunocompromised by either inherited

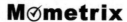
disease or induced by drug therapy. Irradiated components expire at the original outdate or 28 days after radiation occurs, whichever is first.

BLOOD BANK REGULATIONS

OSHA and state regulations outline the requirements for **disposition of blood bags and patient samples**. Blood disposition must comply with OSHA's Bloodborne Pathogen's Standard (29 CFR 1910.1030), which covers blood (semi-liquid, liquid, dried) in containers, in other waste products, or on items, such as sharps. As a regulated waste, the blood must be placed in a container that is closable, leak-proof, labeled (proper color-coding), and closed before removal to avoid any spillage or loss of contents during transport to disposal site.

Temperatures: Blood bank refrigerators are maintained at 2–4 °C with audible and visible alarm if the temperature increases to 6 °C. Freezers are maintained at -20 °C, with alerts when the temperature increases to -19 °C. Incubators usually provide for a range of temperatures (5–70 °C) with much incubation done at 37 °C. The alarm system for refrigerators, freezers, and incubators should be battery powered so it still functions if the electrical supply is cut.

LABEL REQUIREMENTS FOR ALL DONATED BLOOD PRODUCTS

Donated blood products must have a label with the following information: contents; amount of blood collected; volume of blood collected; expiration date; unique number for that particular donated unit; ABO and D type of the blood component; donor classification; prescription requirements; warning regarding infectious agents; FDA license number; information regarding the Circular of Information; type and amount of anticoagulant; and recommended storage temperature.

BLOOD LABELING REQUIREMENTS

The FDA requires that all blood products and materials used for transfusion be labeled with machine-readable **labeling language** to decrease incidence of errors related to the wrong patient or wrong product. The label must contain at least the unique facility ID, the donor's lot number, the product code, and the blood type of the donor. The two labeling languages in use include:

- **Codabar**: Labeling that includes an identifying barcode, a description of the contents (such as "RED BLOOD CELLS"), the volume, additives, storage requirements, and test results of FDA required tests (such as HIV and HBV.
- **ISB-128**: The international standard for identification and labeling as well as transfer of information about body products, including blood. ISB-128 provides a standard terminology, reference tables to apply the appropriate codes, data structures, delivery mechanisms, and standard layout for labels.

EXAMPLE SITUATIONS WHERE TRANSFUSIONS WOULD BE INDICATED

Component	Situations
Red blood cells	Before surgery, radiation therapy, or chemotherapy After trauma For sickle cell anemia For premature infants
Platelets	During excessive post operation bleeding During chemotherapy After a bone marrow transplant
Plasma	Liver disease coupled with bleeding Abnormal coagulation reaction after transfusion Before surgery for those taking anticoagulant drugs

46

Component	Situations
Whole blood	Individuals who have lost 25% or more blood volume Exchange transfusion
Washed red blood cells	Infant and intrauterine transfusions For individuals who suffer anaphylactic, allergic, or febrile reactions to donated plasma proteins
Leukocyte-reduced red blood cells	Chronically transfused patients
Irradiated red blood cells	Bone marrow transplants, progenitor cell transplants, during chemotherapy or radiation therapy, and during intrauterine transfusions Occasionally given to immunodeficient individuals or premature infants

TRANSFUSION TRIGGERS
RED BLOOD CELLS

Hgb (g/dL)	Condition	Transfusions
<6	---	In almost all circumstances
6–7	---	In most circumstances
7	Septic shock >6 hours	Generally indicated
8	Septic shock <6 hours	Generally indicated
7–8	Cardiac or orthopedic surgery	May be indicated, depending on condition
8–10	Oncologic or hematologic-associated thrombocytopenia, acute coronary artery syndrome, continuing bleeding	May be indicated, depending on condition and risks
>10	---	Usually not indicated

CRYOPRECIPITATE

- Adults: Surgical bleeding, severe hemorrhage, post-cardiac surgery hemorrhage.
- Neonates: Factor VIII, XIII deficiencies, von Willebrand disease, congenital fibrinogen deficiency.

FRESH FROZEN PLASMA TRANSFUSION TRIGGERS

Fresh frozen plasma triggers depend on underlying condition:

- Acute DIC
- Bleeding while receiving massive transfusion
- Reversal of warfarin with intracranial hemorrhage
- Fluid for apheresis replacement for TTP and HUS
- Preprocedural prophylactic for those on warfarin if surgery is emergent

PLATELETS TRANSFUSION TRIGGERS

Platelet transfusion triggers depend on age and underlying condition:

	Condition	Platelet Count
Neonate	---	<20,000
	Active bleeding or undergoing invasive procedure	20,000–30,000
	Low birth weight, cerebral hemorrhage, sepsis, thrombocytopenia, coagulation disorders	30,000–50,000

	Condition	Platelet Count
Adult	Not actively bleeding but to undergo major surgery	≤50,000
	Not actively bleeding but to undergo neurological or ocular surgery	≤100,000
	Active bleeding and to undergo surgery	<50,000
	Not actively bleeding and stable	<10,000
	Not actively bleeding and stable but temperature elevated (>38 °C) or to undergo invasive procedure	<20,000

TRANSFUSION-TRANSMITTED INFECTIONS

Viruses	Bacteria	Parasites
Hepatitis A virus (rare)	*Staphylococcus aureus*	Malaria (*Plasmodium* spp.)
Hepatitis B virus	*Anaplasma phagocytophilum*	Chagas (*Trypanosoma cruzi*)
Hepatitis C virus	*Rickettsia rickettsii.*	Babesiosis (*Babesia microti*)
Hepatitis E virus (rare)	*Yersinia enterocolitica*	Leishmaniasis (*Leishmania*
Human immunodeficiency	*Escherichia coli*	*donovani*)
virus (HIV)	*Klebsiella, Proteus, Acinetobacter*	
Human T lymphotropic virus		
West Nile virus		
Cytomegalovirus		**Prion**
Human herpesvirus 8		Variant Creutzfeldt-Jacob
Parvovirus B19		disease (CJD)
SARS-CoV virus		
H5N1 influenza virus		
Dengue virus (DENV)		
Zika virus (ZIKV)		
Chikungunya virus (CHIKV)		

TRANSFUSION REACTIONS

An **anaphylactic** transfusion reaction begins almost immediately after a transfusion is initiated. This is a kind of allergic reaction that manifests with bronchospasms, wheezing, and cough, but no fever. Anaphylactic transfusion reaction can be fatal if not treated immediately. It is caused by a genetic deficiency in IgA antibodies.

A **delayed hemolytic** transfusion reaction typically occurs five to seven days after the transfusion. Symptoms may include fever or mild jaundice. This kind of transfusion reaction is slightly more common than acute hemolytic transfusion reaction, but does not usually pose a threat to survival. The following laboratory tests indicate a possible delayed hemolytic transfusion reaction: positive antibody screen post-transfusion; positive direct antiglobulin test; decreased level of hematocrit; and decreased level of hemoglobin.

An **acute hemolytic** transfusion reaction happens immediately after the transfusion. Possible symptoms include fever, tachycardia, hemoglobinemia, hypotension, and chills. This severe reaction may be the result of incompatible transfusions or reactions between antibodies and antigens. Although acute hemolytic transfusion reactions are quite rare, they are potentially deadly. The following are indications that such a reaction may be occurring: decreased haptoglobin, elevated bilirubin, and elevated plasma free hemoglobin.

Immune-mediated nonhemolytic transfusion reactions occur when the recipient has HLA antibodies that react to the donor's antigens and cytokines. This condition manifests in back pain, headache, nausea, vomiting, and a fever beginning age to 24 hours after the transfusion. This condition is especially common in women who have undergone multiple pregnancies or other individuals who have undergone multiple transfusions. This condition occurs in approximately 1 out of every 200 donor units.

GRAFT VERSUS HOST DISEASE

Graft versus host disease is a rare condition that occurs when T cells from a donor react to the cells of the recipient. This condition typically emerges between 3 and 30 days after the transfusion and may manifest as abnormal liver function, erythromatous maculopapular rash, and fever. Sepsis and even death can result from untreated graft versus host disease.

LOOK-BACK/RECALL PROCEDURES FOR BLOOD PRODUCTS

Look-back procedures are triggered when a transfusion recipient becomes infected and all donors are traced or a donor is discovered to have an infection and all recipients are traced. For donors who convert to positive for HIV, recipients of any component within the previous 12 months must be notified by the hospital or physician. For donors who convert to positive for hepatitis C virus, the recipient or physician must be notified. The physician can make the decision about notifying the recipient. **Recall of blood products** occurs when additional information becomes available about the donor, but in many cases the products have already been transfused and the recipients must be located. The FDA issues recalls and specific directions for look-back, such as the look-back time period. Recall classifications include:

- Class I: Adverse health consequences or death likely.
- Class II: Temporary or reversible adverse health consequences may occur.
- Class III: Very little risk of adverse health consequences.

STEPS TO TAKE BEFORE STARTING A TRANSFUSION AND IF A TRANSFUSION REACTION IS SUSPECTED

Before a transfusion is begun, the lab technician should double-check the tag on the blood bag as well as the paperwork associated with the requisition. During a blood transfusion, the individual's vital signs should be checked every quarter hour. Vital signs that must be checked include body temperature, pulse, blood pressure, and respiration. If a transfusion reaction begins or is suspected, the transfusion should stop immediately. The patient's physician should then be notified.

> **Review Video: Blood Transfusions**
> Visit mometrix.com/academy and enter code: 759682

TRANSFUSION REACTION INVESTIGATION

Transfusion reaction investigations are carried out in response to acute transfusion reactions (mild to severe), delayed, and suspected reactions. The procedure for transfusion reaction investigation includes:

1. Obtain clotted and anticoagulated post-transfusion blood samples for the blood bank/center.
2. Take blood product, transfusion set, and IV solution to blood bank/center.
3. Review labels, IV fluid (saline), pre-and post-transfusion samples, records, and test results.
4. Visually check blood product for signs of contamination and/or hemolysis (note color change) and compare with pre-transfusion samples.

5. Note evidence of post-transfusion plasma hemoglobin and hemoglobinuria.
6. Culture blood product.
7. Conduct patient laboratory investigation: leukocyte count, BNP, HLA class I and II antigens.
8. Obtain first urine sample after reaction and then a 24-hour sample.
9. Repeat blood typing (ABO Rh[D]) to ensure the product was labeled correctly and administered to the correct patient.
10. Compare results of post-transfusion blood typing with pre-transfusion typing and repeat of the procedure if disparities are evident.

Based on the results of the investigation, if an error occurred, the staff must be educated about the error and procedures instituted to avoid further errors.

Blood Banking Practices

PURPOSE AND CRITERIA FOR THERAPEUTIC PHLEBOTOMY

Therapeutic phlebotomy, a blood draw to treat disease, is commonly done to reduce concentration or numbers of red blood cells, ferritin (iron), or porphyrins in the blood for patients with:

- Polycythemia: Increased hemoglobin and hematocrit because of increased red blood cell count that makes blood more viscous.
- Hematochromatosis: Abnormal accumulation of iron in the body, leading to organ damage.
- Porphyrias: Group of disorders in which porphyrins (which are necessary for hemoglobin to function properly) build up in the body.

Blood, usually in about 500 mL units, is withdrawn in a similar manner to blood donations, but most blood is discarded although the FDA allows blood obtained through therapeutic phlebotomy for hematochromatosis to be donated. Patients will have therapeutic phlebotomy on a schedule ordered by the physician, usually to achieve a target hemoglobin. Some patients require blood draws every few days and others once monthly or less frequently.

COMPONENT THERAPY

Component therapy is the practice of transfusing individual blood component products instead of whole blood. This therapeutic method allows for the treatment of a specific deficiency in recipients, while preventing volume overload or a reaction to unnecessary products. Indications for transfusion are specific to each component and are determined in correlation with clinical signs and symptoms.

REGULATION PARAMETERS FOR COMPUTER CROSSMATCH

Under 21 CFR 6096.15 (c), the FDA has established regulations for recipient-donor **computer crossmatch** for transfusions:

- User must be able to verify and accept or reject data.
- Data elements must include the recipient's unique ID number, RBC antibody screening, ABO/Rh (D) typing, sample, and special transfusion requirements (such as leukoreduction) and the donor's unique identification number, component name, ABO/Rh (D) blood type, special requirements and RBC antibody screening.
- Written procedures should outline decision tables and decision rules.
- The system should provide warning messages when actions are out of conformance with decision rules.

- User validation tests must be run on all new equipment/processes in the same environment in which they will be utilized and re-validation carried out according to written program.
- Records must be maintained for all compatibility tests, calibration, equipment standardization, and performance checks for at least 10 years.
- Implementation of computer crossmatch or change in procedure as allowed under licensure must be reported to the FDA.
- Unvalidated systems must undergo testing to meet requirements for validation.

SPECIAL REQUIREMENTS OF BLOOD PRODUCTS

Cytomegalovirus (CMV) negative transfusions: Blood is screened for anti-CMV antibodies and labeled as seronegative although this does not completely eliminate the risk that CMV will be transmitted because the donor's blood may contain CMV from a recent infection without showing antibodies. CMV negative blood is provided for patients who are immunocompromised, such as HIV patients, post-splenectomy patients, and donors for or recipients of bone marrow or stem cell transplants. CMV negative blood is also given for seronegative antepartum patients, low birth weight infants of seronegative mothers, and intrauterine transfusions.

Massive transfusions: Transfusions of 10 (trauma definition) or 20 (traditional definition) units in 24 hours (ratio of plasma to RBCs of 1:1 or 1:2+) for treatment of hemorrhage. Massive transfusions are indicated for loss of 50% of blood volume over a 3-hour period.

Baby units: Red blood cells for infants are prescribed in mL rather than units with the usual volume 5 mL/kg/h (this may be higher with active bleeding) and for platelets 10-20 mL/kg for children up to 15 kg and 300 mL for those over 15 kg.

Microbiology

General Knowledge

BACTERIOLOGY TERMINOLOGY

Mesophilic	Organisms that grow best at moderate temperatures (20–45 °C).
Autotrophic	Self-nourishing organisms that can produce organic constituents from inorganic salts and carbon dioxide.
Semipermeable	Cell membranes that allow the passage of some materials though the membrane but not others.
Ambient	That found in the surroundings, such as ambient light.
Thermophilic	Organisms that grow best at extreme temperatures (41–122 °C).
Heterotopic	Normal cells found in abnormal location or displacement from normal location.
Bacteriophage	Virus that infects and lyses (disintegrates) bacteria.
Pathogenic	Disease-causing organism, such as virus, fungus, and bacterium.
Phagocytosis	Process in which phagocytes engulf other microorganisms, cells, or foreign particles to destroy them.
Bacteria	Single-cell prokaryotic microorganisms that come in a variety of shapes, including coccus (spheres), bacillus (rods), spirals (DNA-like), and filamentous (elongated).
Capsule	The outside polysaccharide layer that surrounds some types of bacteria and protects the cell and provides a virulence factor.
Cytoplasm	Gel-like substance in the interior of the cell that comprises water, enzymes, various nutrients, waste products, and cell structures.
Nucleoid	Strands of DNA found in the cytoplasm.
Cell wall/ membrane	The cell wall is a subcapsular layer composed of peptidoglycan and is rigid to protect the underlying cytoplasmic membrane, which is composed of proteins and phospholipids that regulate the flow of substances to and from the cell. Composition varies among different bacteria. Gram-negative organisms have a thicker outer covering and gram-positive organisms have a thinner outer layer.
Spore	Resistant resting and/or reproductive stage of bacteria.
Flagella	Tail-like structure that helps control movement.
Pili	Hair-like projections that help bacteria attach to different surfaces, such as cells.
Facultative aerobic	Organism that prefers an environment without oxygen but has adapted to survive in the presence of oxygen. Examples include *Staphylococcus* spp. and *Lactobacillus*.
Microaerophilic aerobe	Organism that needs lower levels of oxygen than that typically found in the environment to survive and may also require higher levels of carbon dioxide. Examples include *Campylobacter* spp. and *Helicobacter pylori*.
Aerobic	Organism that lives and reproduces in an environment with oxygen. Obligate aerobes can only live in oxygenated environments. Example includes *Pseudomonas aeruginosa*.

52

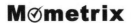

Facultative anaerobic	Organism that is able to live and reproduce in an environment with or without oxygen. Examples include *Escherichia coli* and *Streptococcus* spp.
Anaerobic	Organism that lives and reproduces in an environment without oxygen. Obligate anaerobes can only live in the absence of oxygen. Example includes *Clostridium botulinum.*

GRAM'S METHOD OF STAINING BACTERIA

Gram staining method is used to distinguish between gram-positive and gram-negative bacteria in the laboratory. Stain the sample with crystal violet. Next, treat the sample with a solution of iodine. Add alcohol or another organic solvent to the sample. Examine the sample under the microscope. Gram-positive bacteria will still be stained a violet/blue color. Gram-negative bacteria, however, will be colorless. In order to make the gram-negative bacteria stand out, counterstain the sample with safrinin. This counterstain will make the gram-negative bacteria appear red in color, and the gram-positive bacteria will still appear violet/blue in color.

GRAM-POSITIVE BACTERIA VS. GRAM NEGATIVE BACTERIA STAIN RETENTION

In the Gram test, gram-positive bacteria will retain their bluish/violet color from the crystal violet stain even after being treated with an organic solvent. Gram-negative bacteria, on the other hand, will lose their color and appear colorless after being treated with an organic solvent. Gram-negative bacteria have a very thin cell wall, so when they are washed with the alcohol, the stain is liberated from the bacteria. Gram-positive bacteria, on the other hand, have a very thick cell wall made of peptidoglycan, so the alcohol solvent is not able to liberate the violet stain from the bacteria.

USES OF VARIOUS STAINS IN THE LABORATORY

Crystal violet is used for the gram staining of bacterial cell walls. Gram-negative bacteria will appear red or pink in color, and gram-positive bacteria will appear dark blue or violet in color when treated with crystal violet.

Wright's stain is used to help distinguish blood cells. It can be used with either blood or bone marrow samples. Often it is used when performing white blood cell (WBC) counts if infections are expected in the patient.

Sudan black B is a stain that is used to identify the presence of triglycerides or lipids. Sudan black B will stain these compounds a bluish-black color.

Giemsa stain is a stain that can be used to identify bacteria and other parasites. Giemsa stain can be used with blood films, blood smears, or bone marrow samples. Giemsa stain will stain parasites or bacterial cells a purple color, while the human cells will be colored pink. Giemsa stain is made of a combination of eosin and methylene blue.

ACID-FAST STAIN

The acid-fast stain, also called the **Ziehl–Neelsen** stain, is performed to detect organisms that cause tuberculosis. These bacteria are deemed acid-fast bacilli (**AFB**) due to their ability to be visualized by the acid-fast staining process. This is a differential stain for mycobacterium that will retain the primary stain, whereas all other bacteria, without a cell wall containing mycolic acid, will decolorize and counterstain.

The acid-fast procedure consists of the primary stain, carbolfuchsin, with heat to facilitate penetration of the stain into the cell walls of mycobacterium with high lipid content. A 3% hydrochloric acid, 97% ETOH decolorizer is then used to leach the primary stain from the cell walls of bacteria that do not contain high contents of mycolic acid. Methylene blue is used as a counterstain to make all of the other bacteria a visible blue color.

Acid-fast/Ziehl–Neelsen procedure:

1. Heat fix stain/slide for 2 hours at 65–70 °C or 15 minutes at 80 °C.
1. Flood stain with heated carbolfuchsin at 60 °C for 5 minutes.
2. Rinse with water.
3. Decolorize with 3% HCl/97% ETOH ~2 minutes (for an average-thickness slide).
4. Rinse with water.
5. Flood with methylene blue 1–3 minutes.
6. Rinse with water.
7. Allow to air dry.
8. Examine under an oil immersion lens.

Interpretation:

- Mycobacterium (AFB) will stain red.
- All other bacteria will stain blue.

MODIFIED ACID-FAST STAIN

The modified acid-fast stain, or **Kinyoun** stain, is performed to detect organisms that cause tuberculosis by differentiating **AFB** from all other bacteria in a microbiology specimen. This achieves the same outcome as the acid-fast stain, without the use of heat. The modification of heat requirements means that the Kinyoun stain is also referred to as "cold" acid-fast staining.

This method uses a carbolfuchsin stain prepared with phenol to facilitate the penetration of stain into the lipid-rich cell walls of mycobacteria. An acid/alcohol solution, comprised of 3% HCl and 97% ETOH, is used to decolorize nonmycobacterium organisms by removing the primary stain from their cell walls. A counterstain of methylene blue or malachite green is used to allow decolorized bacteria to become visible again upon examination, allowing for differentiation to occur.

Modified acid-fast/Kinyoun procedure:

1. Heat fix stain/slide for 2 hours at 65–70 °C or 15 minutes at 80 °C.
2. Flood stain with Kinyoun carbolfuchsin at room temperature for 5 minutes.
3. Rinse with water.
4. Decolorize with 3% HCl/97% ETOH for ~2 minutes (for an average-thickness slide).
5. Rinse with water.
6. Flood with methylene blue or malachite green for 1–3 minutes.
7. Rinse with water.
8. Allow to air dry.
9. Examine under an oil immersion lens.

Interpretation:

- Mycobacterium (AFB): red
- All other bacteria: blue (methylene blue) or green (malachite green).

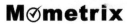

GIEMSA STAIN

Giemsa stain is used in the visualization, differentiation, and identification of parasites in clinical specimens. Most commonly, Giemsa stains are performed on blood smears, but they may be performed on specimens from other sources as well, such as lesion biopsies and various aspirates. Thin-film smears allow for RBC inclusion and extracellular morphologies to be more easily observed, whereas thick smears allow a larger volume of sample to be surveyed for potential parasites. Giemsa-stained blood films are used as diagnostic testing for malarial infections, due to the *Babesia* parasite present demonstrating the characteristic "Maltese cross" ring formation.

Prepared from a powder containing azure, methylene blue, eosin dye, and methanol, Giemsa stock stain is diluted with buffered water to properly stain slides for observation. In blood smears, the Giemsa stain color in parasites will mimic the color of the stained WBCs. This acts as an internal quality control for the method. The morphologic characteristics of parasites observed with this stain are used for differentiation and subsequent identification.

Giemsa stain procedure:

1. Place a slide into absolute methanol for 30 seconds to fix a thin sample to the slide. (Skip this step for thick slides; methanol fixation is not needed.)
2. Allow the slide to air dry.
3. Place the slide in 1 part Giemsa stock stain to 20 parts buffered water for 20 minutes*.
4. Remove the slide and drain off the excess stain.
5. Dip the slide in buffered water one to two times to wash the slide.
6. Remove the slide and allow it to air dry, propped in a vertical position.
7. Observe the slide under a 40× lens and then under an immersion lens with a light microscope.

*Dilutions of Giemsa stock stain may vary between 10 and 50, depending on the preparation. The staining time must be adjusted for the different stain concentration present. Typically, the dilution factor will correspond to the appropriate duration of staining (e.g., 1:10, 10 minutes; 1:30, 30 minutes).

Outcome:

- Parasitic forms: blue to purple with reddish nuclei
- RBCs: pale gray-blue
- WBC nucleus, cytoplasm: purple, pale-purple, respectively
- Eosinophilic granules: bright purple-red
- Neutrophilic granules: deep pink-purple.

ACRIDINE ORANGE

Fluorochrome acridine orange is a nonspecific stain that binds to nucleic acids. This stain is used to confirm the presence of bacteria in blood culture smears in the following instances: the Gram stain is difficult to interpret, the presence of bacteria is highly suspected but not observed via light microscopy, or for the detection of bacteria incapable of retaining Gram stains, such as mycoplasmas.

Acridine Orange Procedure:

1. Fix a blood culture smear to a glass slide with heat or methanol.
2. Flood the slide with acridine orange, allowing the stain to remain on the slide for two minutes without drying.
3. Rinse the slide with tap water and allow to air dry.
4. Examine under ultraviolet fluorescent microscopy.

Interpretation:

Any bacteria or host cells present will fluoresce bright orange against a dark or green-fluorescing background.

INTERPRETING/IDENTIFYING STRUCTURES THROUGH MICROBIOLOGICAL SLIDE PREPARATIONS

Direct (wet mount)	Because the organism is not fixed, motile organisms (such as *Vibrio*) and fragile organisms (such as those with filaments or sporulating bodies) are more easily identified. Wet mount is used for fecal examination for O & P. Dark-field microscopy helps to identify spirochetes, and India ink preparation, *C. neoformans*.
Direct (dry mount)	The organisms are killed, hardened, and adhered to the slide so they can't change shape or configuration. Simple staining (crystal violet, methylene blue [most commonly used], safranin, carbol-fuchsin) helps to identify gross morphology and to differentiate types of organisms. Gram-staining helps to differentiate Gram-positive from Gram-negative pathogens. Gram-staining also helps to determine the type of biochemical tests or culture media to use. Acid fast staining is used primarily to identify *Mycobacterium tuberculosis* and *M. leprae*. Ziehl-Neelsen hot staining utilizes carbol-fuchsin solution to diagnose *M. tuberculosis* from sputum sample.

Media Quality Control, Techniques, and Cultures

BACTERIAL CULTURE METHODS
DIFFERENT MEDIA
A number of different media are utilized for bacterial cultures, which are used to increase the numbers of a microorganism, select specific types, or differentiate them:

- **Differential**: The media changes in appearance with color change as a biochemical reaction to different bacteria, helping to distinguish different organisms.
- **Selective**: The media encourages the growth of one type of microorganism while inhibiting the growth of others.
- **Enrichment**: Media enriched with additives (such as sheep's blood) that encourages the growth of a specific type of microorganism.
- **Candle jar**: Inoculated specimen plates are placed inside of a glass jar and a small candle placed on top of the upper plate. As the candle burns, it uses up most of the oxygen and the carbon dioxide stimulates anaerobic bacterial growth although some aerobic growth may also occur because of residual oxygen.
- **Living host cells**: Used for some specific types of microorganisms that only grow in living cells, such as some leprosy.

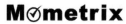

ANAEROBIC MEDIA

Anaerobic microorganisms are most often found in abscesses and deep wounds, such as bites, blood, and cerebrospinal fluid. Aseptic technique is especially important to avoid contamination, and cotton swabs should not be used to collect a specimen because they may damage the microorganisms. Sample must be transported in an oxygen-free container.

- **Anaerobic media**: Pre-reduced anaerobically sterilized (PRAS) media is available, but is expensive and other media (selective, differential, or enriched) may be utilized as well if processed properly.
- **Anaerobic techniques**: Inoculated specimen plates are placed inside an anaerobic jar with an inlet and outlet and an electrified catalyst combines hydrogen and oxygen to provide anaerobic environment. With the gas pack, the inoculated plates are placed inside a container and water added combine hydrogen and oxygen, producing an anaerobic environment. Methylene blue is utilized as an anaerobic indicator.

MacConkey Agar

MacConkey agar is a medium used in the laboratory to grow mycobacteria, such as *Mycobacteria chelonei*, and to differentiate between different types of mycobacteria. It is also used to stain gram negative bacteria for lactose fermentation. MacConkey agar consists of lactose, peptone, bile salts, crystal violet dye, and a neutral red dye. The red dye is what stains the bacteria that are fermenting the lactose present in the agar. MacConkey agar is used to not only identify various fast-growing mycobacteria, but it can be used to identify other pathogens, such as *Salmonella* and *Shigella*.

Additives Used in Media Preparation

Media for culture must allow microorganisms to grow and reproduce, so various additives (nutrients or inhibitors) are added to an aqueous base to create different types of media. **Complex media**, which usually contain glucose and animal or plant proteins (protein hydrolysates such as tryptone), support various types of heterotrophic microorganisms. **Defined media** have exact percentages of various additives (such as mineral salts, growth factors, and simple carbohydrate) and support specific microorganisms and are generally required for microbiological assays. **Selective media** often have additives (such as mannitol) to suppress growth of undesirable microorganisms while promoting growth of others (such as *Staphylococcus aureus)*. **Differential media** have additives that help to distinguish different types of colonies. **Enriched media** contains additives (such as sheep blood or heated blood [chocolate]) to encourage increased growth of specific microorganisms. Commonly used additives include arginine, biotin, dextrin, galactose, glucose, lactose, mannitol, citric acid, sorbitol, and EDTA.

BACTERIOSTATIC

A drug that is bacteriostatic is one that limits the reproduction and growth of new bacteria. Bacteriostatic antibiotics can do this by negatively affecting the cellular metabolism of bacteria. They also can hamper the production of the bacteria's DNA and protein. All of these interferences by the bacteriostatic drug have an effect on the growth and development of new bacteria. Some examples of bacteriostatic antibiotics are: Lincosamides, sulphonamides, tetracycline, and macrolides. Bacteriostatic antibiotics should be distinguished from bactericidal antibiotics, in that bactericidal antibiotics actually kill bacteria, whereas bacteriostatic antibiotics only curtail their reproduction. An example of bactericidal antibiotic is penicillin.

ANTIMICROBIAL AGENT EXAMPLES

Gentamicin works by interfering with protein synthesis. Gentamicin can be used to treat urinary tract infections.

Vancomycin works by interfering with the synthesis of bacterial cell walls. Vancomycin can be used to treat serious respiratory infections in patients that are allergic to penicillins.

Clindamycin works by interfering with protein synthesis. Clindamycin can be used to treat respiratory infections.

Rifampin works by interfering with the synthesis of bacterial ribonucleic acid (RNA). Rifampin is used to treat tuberculosis.

Penicillin works by interfering with the synthesis of bacterial cell walls. Penicillin can be used to treat pneumonia.

Tetracycline works by interfering with the synthesis of bacterial RNA. It can be used to treat infections of the respiratory tract.

SPECIMEN COLLECTION, PREPARATION, AND REJECTION CRITERIA

Specimens must be obtained following established protocols and in the proper tube or container with the correct additive, such as sodium citrate in a blood specimen. The specimen must be stored and/or transported in a manner appropriate to the type of specimen. **Rejection criteria** may vary according to the type of specimen and test, and specimens are generally not discarded until the ordering healthcare provider is notified. Rejection criteria may include:

- Incorrect tube or container.
- Incorrect or missing requisition/order.
- Specimen size insufficient for testing.
- Hemolysis evident.
- Specimen not correctly labeled.
- Tube/container leaking or contaminated with body fluids. (Note: critical specimens may be salvaged after tube/container thoroughly cleansed with 10% hypochlorite [bleach] solution.)
- Specimen contained in syringe with attached needle.
- Date/Collection time not noted on specimen.
- Specimen too old for testing.
- Specimen improperly stored/transported.

CULTURING CLINICAL SPECIMENS

Blood	Obtain two (anaerobic and aerobic) 8–10 mL specimens at temperature peak and/or multiple at 30-minute to 1-hour intervals and inoculate the blood culture vials. Incubate and monitor as per protocol. Gram stain samples from positive cultures and subculture for aerobic (sheep blood, chocolate agar) and anaerobic organisms according to protocol (usually after 18–48 hours). Incubate at 35–37 °C for up to 7 days and inspect at least 2 times daily.
Urine	Obtain clean catch or catheterized specimen in sterile container. Process immediately or store specimen at 4 °C. Prepare a slide for gram staining with one drop of mixed (not centrifuged) urine and examine under microscope or conduct the leukocyte esterase strip test. Negative findings generally indicate culture is unnecessary, but positive findings should be followed by inoculation of a MacConkey agar plate with incubation at 35–37°C for 24–48 hours.

Stool	Collect specimen prior to beginning antibiotics in a sterile container or use cotton-tipped swab inserted into the rectum and rotated to obtain a fecal sample. Insert swab into sterile tube. The specimen should be processed as soon as possible or stored at 4 °C. Specimen should be examined microscopically and plates inoculated. A fecal suspension with saline may be necessary for swabs or solid stool specimens if multiple plates must be inoculated. This also helps eliminate organic matter. Various types of agar may be used depending on the suspected organisms. Incubate at 35–37 °C for 24–48 hours.
Sputum	Collect sputum specimen in wide-mouthed sterile container and process within one hour. Record macroscopic appearance and prepare a gram-stain for microscopic examination. If fewer than 10 PMNs are noted per epithelial cells, the specimen should be rejected. If more, agar plates (various types) should be inoculated and incubated 35–37 °C for 24–48 hours (inspect after 18 hours).
Throat (upper respiratory)	Collect 2 specimens with sterile swabs rubbed over the back of the throat and tonsillar areas, avoiding the tongue and other structures, and place in sterile tube for transfer. Process within 4 hours or place in transport medium. Gram-staining is generally done only on specific request. Inoculate a blood agar (low glucose) by rubbing the swab over 1 quadrant and streak the remaining quadrants with a sterile loop. Place a bacitracin disk and a co-trimoxazole disk over the streaked area to aid in identification of bacteria. Incubate at 35–37 °C for 18 hours and inspect for colonies and then inspect again at 48 hours. Gram-stain colony samples to aid in identification.
Cerebrospinal fluid	Collect 5–10 mL CSF in 2 sterile tubes and process immediately. The CSF should be assessed macroscopically and microscopically through direct microscopy, gram-stain, and acid-fast stain. Inoculate plates appropriate to bacteria identified through microscopy or multiple media if unclear and incubate for at least 3 days with temperature and conditions determined by the type of agar and environment required for suspected organisms (aerobic, anaerobic).
Wound	Collect specimen through aspiration (preferred) of exudate or tissue sample or by wiping the wound with 2 cotton swabs and placing swabs in sterile container, in transport medium if processing cannot be done immediately. The exudate should be examined with direct, Gram-stain, and acid-fast stain microscopy and macroscopically (color, consistency, odor). Depending on results of the microscopic examination, various types of plates (minimum 3) should be inoculated. If using a swab for inoculation, wipe the swab across one quadrant of a plate and streak the remaining quadrants with a wire loop. Incubation time, temperature, and environment depend on the type of plate and the suspected organisms.
Abscess	Similar to wound culture although aspirant only is generally used. Organisms may be polymicrobial, including both aerobic and anaerobic bacteria, depending on the site of the abscess. Culturing for anaerobic bacteria (both gram-negative and gram-positive) should always be included, so the specimen must be protected from exposure to oxygen and incubation done at 35 °C for 48 hours and then examined.

Genital fluids	Females: Collect specimen with pelvic examination and speculum moistened only with water. Wipe away mucus about the cervix with a cotton swab/ball and discard. Then insert a cotton swab and wipe the vaginal posterior fornix for the first sample, use another swab to collect an endocervical sample by inserting the swab into the cervix and rotating it for 10 seconds. Males: Collect oropharyngeal, urethral, anorectal specimens in a similar manner, inserting swab 3–4 cm inside urethra and 4–5 cm inside anus/rectum. Examination: Examine macroscopically for color and odor and through direct and gram-stain microscopy. Culturing should be done to identify *Neisseria gonorrhoeae* (especially in females) with direct inoculation of Thayer-Martin agar incubated at 35 °C in candle-jar environment for 48 hours (checked daily for colonies).
Ear exudates	Collect specimens with two swabs inserted gently into the ear canal and rotated. Examine through direct and Gram-stain microscopy. Culture is usually carried out on MacConkey medium, blood agar, and Sabouraud dextrose medium with antibiotics, depending on the type of bacteria observed through microscopy with temperature and environment also dependent on suspected bacteria.
Eye exudate	Collect 2 specimens with a sterile cotton swab from the lower conjunctival sac and from the inner canthus of each eye and place in sterile tubes. Examine (first swabs) through direct, Gram-stain, and Giemsa stain microscopically and then carry out cultures (second swabs). Volume of bacteria for both ear and eye exudates tends to be low, so antibiotic disks are generally not used. Media commonly used includes MacConkey agar (under aerobic condition), blood agar (candle jar), and chocolate agar (candle jar). Incubate 18–24 hours, examine, and incubate another 48 hours if necessary.
Tissue	Collect specimens through surgical procedure or endoscopy and place in sterile container in transport medium. Examine macroscopically and microscopically. Process the tissue sample as per protocol for type of tissue and inoculate various types of culture media, depending on the tissue type and suspected microorganisms. Incubate at 35–37 °C for times indicated for media.
IV catheter tips	Collect the IV catheter intact and transport in sterile container. Cut a 5 cm section from the catheter tip and roll that four times over a solid medium plate or immerse the section in broth culture medium. Incubate at 35–37 °C for the times indicated for media and examine for colonies (>15 significant). Various other methods may be utilized, and blood cultures are usually done simultaneously.
IUD	Similar to procedures for IV catheter tips. Endocervical (and sometimes blood) cultures are usually done simultaneously.

CONTINUOUS BLOOD CULTURE MONITORING SYSTEMS

Blood culture monitoring systems continuously assess blood culture bottles for the presence of bacterial growth. Cultures are incubated at 35–37 °C for 5 to 7 days in a chamber that is constantly rocking to promote the growth of any potential pathogens that are present. Gas sensors in the chamber use fluorescence to detect any CO_2 production within the blood culture bottles. The CO_2 gas production, turbidity, lysis of RBCs, and visual observation of bacterial colonies in a blood culture bottle are indicative of bacterial growth. If bacterial growth is detected, the system will alarm to notify lab staff that the presumptively positive blood culture bottle should be subcultured and Gram stained for organism detection and identification.

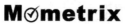

Continuous monitoring systems are advantageous because they monitor bacterial growth without the need to visually inspect bottles each day or blindly subculture and Gram stain every blood culture collected. Monitoring systems can also be interfaced with laboratory information systems (LIS) to allow for easier reporting of results and for reducing the risk of clerical errors.

DIRECT AND MOLECULAR METHODS USED IN DETECTION OF CSF INFECTIONS

Direct detection methods for the evaluation and diagnosis of CSF infections includes stains, rapid latex antigen testing, and serological testing. Bacterial meningitis can be detected by the presence of bacteria found on a Gram stain. India ink and acid-fast stain preparations allow for the direct detection of *Cryptococcus* and tuberculosis pathogens, respectively. Rapid latex antigen tests are useful in the immediate detection of classic meningitis causing bacteria such as *S. pneumoniae, H. influenzae,* group B strep, *E. coli, Neisseria meningitides,* and *Cryptococcus neoformans.* Latex beads coated with sensitized monoclonal IgG antibodies for each bacterium are added to a test card with a CSF sample, mixed, and mechanically rotated for 5 minutes. Agglutination of the latex determines the presence of bacterial antigens, thus indicating a bacterial infection. Serological methods are also used in determining syphilis infections of the CNS. The fluorescent treponemal antibody absorption test is very sensitive but less specific in CSF samples than serum. Molecular methods aid in detecting pathogens that do not grow on routine media or in patients who have already had antibiotic treatments. PCR testing is available for the detection and amplification of nucleic acids in the RNA or DNA of various CSF pathogens including bacteria, virus, fungi, and parasites.

COLONY MORPHOLOGY ON MICROBIOLOGY CULTURES

A bacterial colony is a visible mass of identical organisms that grows from a single bacterial cell. Different genera, species, and strains of bacteria present with distinct visual appearances that are used as the first step in isolating and identifying infectious agents. Evaluating colony morphology also aids in determining the purity of a culture by more easily recognizing contamination of other organisms. Within 18–24 hours after being inoculated with sample, organisms growing on microbiology media are visually observed. A hand lens or magnifying glass can be used to aid in identifying key characteristics. Colony morphology is evaluated by the following characteristics:

- Colony size
- Form and margins
- Surface features, texture, and consistency
- Elevation
- Color, transparency, and iridescence.

CATEGORIZATION AND INTERPRETATION OF COLONY MORPHOLOGY CHARACTERISTICS

Colony morphology is categorized by size, form, margins, and elevation characteristics in the following ways:

- **Colony size** is categorized by diameter:
  - Pinpoint or punctiform < 1 mm
  - Small 1–2 mm
  - Medium 3–4 mm
  - Large > 5 mm
- **Forms** are categorized as
  - Circular, symmetrical circle
  - Irregular, lacking symmetry

- o Filamentous, exhibiting threadlike branching
- o Rhizoid, exhibiting a branching, rootlike shape
- The **margins**, or edges, of a colony are most commonly evaluated as
  - o Entire, meaning smooth
  - o Undulate, meaning wavy
  - o Lobular, fingerlike growth spreading outward
  - o Scalloped, rounded projections resembling a scallop shell
  - o Filiform, thin and wavy layers spreading outward
- The **elevation** of bacterial colonies refers to its cross-sectional shape. Colony elevations are categorized by the following shapes:
  - o Flat
  - o Raised
  - o Convex, curved or rounded upward
  - o Crateriform, sunken in the middle
  - o Umbonate, with the middle protruding upward

Surface texture and consistency are described as having the following characteristics:

- **Textures** are described with the following terms:
  - o Smooth
  - o Wrinkled, shriveled
  - o Rough, granular
  - o Dull, no shine
  - o Glistening, shining
- The **consistency** of colonies is described as the following:
  - o Moist
  - o Dry
  - o Viscid, thick and sticky
  - o Mucoid, moist and sticky
  - o Butyrous, butter-like

Colonies can exhibit a variety of transparencies and pigmentations:

- Colony **transparency** is categorized as
  - o Transparent, clear, see-through
  - o Translucent, semiclear, frosted-glass appearance
  - o Opaque, unable to see through
  - o Iridescent, color changing in reflective light
- Sheep blood and chocolate agars often yield the following **colony colors**:
  - o White
  - o Cream
  - o Yellow
- Differential and selective medias can produce many colors based on the organism's biochemical properties such as:
  - o Pink
  - o Green
  - o Blue
  - o Black

ISOLATING, IDENTIFYING, AND DIFFERENTIATING MICROORGANISMS

Isolating, identifying, and differentiating microorganisms begin with direct examination under a microscope so that the shape, size, cell wall characteristics, and linkages can be noted. This helps to identify the basic type: bacilli, cocci, coccobacilli, and spirals. This is followed by Gram-staining, which helps to differentiate Gram-positive and Gram-negative organisms. Based on these assessments and suspected organism, various media are selected for culturing of the sample because some encourage the growth of certain organisms and others inhibit growth. The cultured plates are incubated to encourage growth of colonies and the colonies examined (size, shape, surface, texture, color) to further identify the organism. In some cases, sub-cultures are required to differentiate species. Additional methods include API® (test strips), biochemical testing, and carbohydrate fermentation tests. If the organism is still not identified, then DNA sequencing may be carried out.

PROCESSING AND PLANTING OF SPECIMENS

INOCULATING AGAR AND BROTH

Always maintain aseptic technique. To inoculate:

- Agar deep: Insert the needle straight to the bottom and withdraw straight.
- Agar plate: Lift one side of the lid and slide the loop in horizontally, streaking the inoculum back and forth on the surface only. Reflame the loop after each third of the plate is streaked, reinoculate, turn the plate 90° and continue until the entire plate (or 3 quadrants) is streaked. Invert plate for incubation.
- Agar slant: Either insert loop to the bottom of the tube and withdraw straight (for growth pattern) or in back-and-forth manner (for increased growth).
- Broth: Swish the loop back and forth about the tube.

Once inoculation is complete, then the plate/tube is placed in the incubator with the temperature and duration determined by the type of medium and the type of organism.

OBTAINING INOCULUM FROM AGAR AND BROTH

Media used for cultures must be sterilized and maintained in sterile conditions and organisms transferred to the media using aseptic transfer techniques. Tube caps are removed and tops heated (up draft) to keep contamination away from the inside. Inoculation is typically made with a sterile inoculating needle (agar deeps) or wire loop (agar plates/broths). The inoculating needle or wire loop must be heated to red hot and cooled before transfer. To obtain inoculum:

- Agar plate: Lift one side of the lid (do not completely uncover) and use the wire loop to lift one colony (or part of a large colony) of the surface.
- Agar slant: Use the wire loop to scrape inoculum from the surface.
- Broth: Mix by shaking slightly and then immerse the loop and withdraw carefully (a film should be noted across the loop).

Note: For agar deep, obtain inoculum with a sterile needle.

NORMAL FLORA

Normal flora are those bacteria (predominate), fungi, and protists that are normally found on the surface tissues, including the skin and the mucous membranes. The most common bacteria are *Staphylococcus epidermidis* and *Staphylococcus aureus*, which are found on both skin and mucous membranes, as is *Streptococcus pyogenes.* Overgrowth of these organisms often results in skin infections, and these bacteria may migrate through open wounds. *Staphylococcus aureus* is a leading cause of infectious diseases. *Streptococcus mitis, salivarius, mutans, pneumoniae,* and *faecalis* are found on mucous membranes but not on the skin. Some bacteria are more common in one area of the body than others. For example, *Escherichia coli* is most common in the lower gastrointestinal tract, so it spreads through the fecal-oral route, and *Neisseria meningitidis* is found in the nose and pharynx, which allows it to spread through droplets.

RECOGNIZING AND IDENTIFYING PATHOGENS FROM CULTURES

Pathogen identification from cultures involves assessing colony morphology. Colonies may be circular, filamentous, rhizoid, or irregular in shape and may have various types of elevation, including flat, raised/rounded, convex, pulvinate, cratered, and knobby (umbonate). The colony margins may also help to identify organisms and may be solid, undulating, lobular/lobate, curled, or filamentous. The surface of the colony may vary according to the organism. Surfaces may, for example, be smooth, rough, granular, or glistening. The texture of the colony may range from dry or brittle to moist or viscous. The color of the colony may vary also depending on the medium and the organism. For example, on MacConkey agar, *Escherichia coli* colonies are pink. Colors may range from colorless, pink, red, blue, green, to black. The diameter (in millimeters) of the colonies varies according to the types of organism, so measuring the colonies can aid in identification.

SPECIMEN SOURCES AND COLLECTION TO CHECK FOR INFECTION IN BLOODSTREAM

To diagnose an infection in the bloodstream, or **sepsis**, the most common samples collected are blood cultures. **Blood cultures** consist of blood being added to aerobic and anerobic bottles containing a broth that supports microbial growth. Ideally, two sets of blood cultures will be collected from separate sites to compare results and more easily determine false positives due to contamination from true-positive results. If infection originating from a port or intravenous catheter is suspected, draw one set of cultures from the port or catheter line and the other set peripherally. Intravenous catheter tips may cause infection from opportunistic skin flora at the time of insertion or removal of the device. After removal, the catheter tip itself may be cultured if it is a suspected source of infection.

The procedure for peripheral collection of blood cultures is as follows:

- At the site chosen to draw, aseptically cleanse the skin in a circular motion with 70% alcohol, and allow it to dry.
- Repeat cleansing of the site with iodine, allow it to dry for 1 minute.
- Following proper phlebotomy practices, insert the needle into the vein and withdraw the blood. Do not change the needle before injecting the blood into the blood culture bottle. The necessary volume for blood culture bottles to achieve a 1:10 dilution of blood to broth is 10 mL for adult aerobic or anaerobic and 5 mL for pediatric patients.
- Repeat the procedure at a second draw site.

TESTING FOR MULTI-DRUG RESISTANT TUBERCULOSIS (MDR-TB)

Testing for multi-drug-resistant tuberculosis (*Mycobacterium tuberculosis*) includes:

- **Agar proportion**: Use Felsin quadrant plates, which contain an antibiotic-impregnated disk in 3 quadrants with the remaining quadrant serving as the control. Molten Middlebrook 7H11 agar medium is poured over the antimicrobial disks and incubated overnight to allow the antibiotic agent to diffuse through the medium. Then each quarter is inoculated and the plate sealed and incubated at 37° C for 3 to 4 weeks. The organism is susceptible to the antibiotic if there is >200 colonies in the control quadrant and none in the antibiotic-containing quadrant.

64

- **96 well microtiter plate (MYCOTB)**: This method requires first growing colonies of the microorganism and then inoculating the wells in the microtiter plate. The plate contains 12 antimicrobial drugs in different concentrations (isoniazid, rifampin, ethambutol, kanamycin, cycloserine, amikacin, moxifloxacin, ofloxacin, rifabutin, streptomycin, ethionamide, and para-aminosalicylic acid. (Note pyrazinamide must be tested for separately because it requires an acidic environment). The plate is incubated for 14 days and the growth in each well is evaluated utilizing a mirror box or a semi-automatic plate reader.

Bacterial Identification

SYSTEMS OF BACTERIAL IDENTIFICATION

Various systems of **bacterial identification** are utilized:

- **API**: Test strips with up to 20 biochemical tests provide 2- to 72-hour (depending on type of organism) identification of gram-negative, gram-positive, anaerobic, and yeast organisms, as well as strips for specific tests (such as carbohydrate metabolism) and organisms (such as *Lactobacillus* and *Bacillus*).
- **Automated**: Software is available for PCR and microarray-based identification systems.
- **Biochemical**: Organisms are identified by adding reagents to a substrate, which results in an enzymatic reaction that causes a color change that can be quantified. Different reagents are utilized to identify specific organisms. For example, TDA reagent is used to identify *Proteus* species.
- **Carbohydrate metabolism** (includes lactose fermentation, sucrose fermentation, glucose fermentation): This method identifies organisms by their ability ferment the carbohydrate. Broth containing lactose, sucrose, or glucose is inoculated with the suspected organism and a color change indicates fermentation is occurring. For example, the glucose fermentation can differentiate different species of *Enterobacteriaceae*.

BACTERIAL DIFFERENTIATING TESTS

Optochin susceptibility test utilizes disks (P) that contain optochin, to which *S. pneumoniae* are susceptible. The disk is placed on top of a blood agar plate covering zone one (area that is heavily inoculated with a specimen) and incubated. If growth is inhibited about the disk, this is an indication that the bacteria are *S. pneumoniae.*

Camp test is used to identify group B strep (particularly *Streptococcus agalactiae)* and gram-positive rods, which produces CAMP factor (extracellular protein) that acts in conjunction with beta-lysin (produced by *Staphylococcus aureus)* to promote hemolysis of sheep RBCs. The test utilizes a sheep blood agar plate, which is inoculated in a line across the plate with *Staphylococcus aureus.* The plate is then inoculated with the test specimen in a straight line perpendicular (2–3 cm in length) to the *Staph* line (at least 1 cm away and not touching it), placed in incubator at 37 °C for 24–28 hours, and then checked to see if hemolysis has occurred from the interaction.

Indole test is used to differentiate Enterobacteriaceae genera (*Escherichia, Proteus, Salmonella, Shigella, Enterobacter)*, which are gram-negative facultative anaerobes that can break down tryptophan into indole. A 4 mL tube of tryptophan broth is inoculated with a sample from an 18- to 24-hour culture. The inoculated tube is then incubated at 37 °C for 24–28 hours. Then 0.5 mL of Kovac's reagent is added to the tube and the color observed. If the sample is positive, a rose to bright red color change will appear in the top reagent layer. **Indole spot test** is used to differentiate indole positive members of a species from indole negative (such as *Klebsiella* pneumoniae (negative) from other *Klebsiella* spp. (positive). A few drops of Indole Spot reagent are placed on filter paper, which is inoculated with a sample of an 18- to 24-hour culture by rubbing the sample over the wet area of the paper. A color change occurs within 3 minutes: blue for positive and pink for negative.

Beta-lactamase (Cefinase) test (discs impregnated with Nitrocefin) is used to identify organisms (anaerobic bacteria, *Staphylococci, Enterococci, N. gonorrhoeae,* and *Haemophilus influenzae,* which produce beta-lactamase. One sample is used for each disk. Place disks on empty Petri dish and place one drop of sterile distilled water on each disk. Inoculate disks with colonies and note change in disk color to yellow or red for positive organisms. Time to reaction varies according to organism:

- 1 minute: H. influenzae, N. gonorrhoeae.
- 5 minutes: Enterococcus faecalis.
- 30 minutes: Anaerobic bacteria.
- 60 minutes: Staphylococcus aureus.

Oxidase test is used to identify aerobic bacteria that produce cytochrome oxidase (an enzyme). A small sample of the organism culture is removed from an agar plate or slant tube (being careful not to include any agar) with a swab and one drop of reagent used to dampen the culture. If the bacteria are aerobic, a positive reaction will cause the dampened swab/culture to turn violet to purple in 10–30 seconds.

Catalase test is used to identify aerobic organisms (*Staphylococcus),* which are usually catalase positive and can release oxygen from hydrogen peroxide, resulting in production of a white froth. This test should not be done on blood agar but rather on samples in slant tubes after 18-24 hours of growth. A few drops of hydrogen peroxide are added to the slant tube and observed for froth reaction. If the results appear negative, a sample can be placed under a microscope and the hydrogen peroxide added to more easily observe the reaction.

Tryptic soy broth (TSB) with NaCl (6.5%) is used to assess whether an organism can live in a high-salt environment. While most organisms die, *Enterococci, Aerococci,* and *Staphylococci* can tolerate the environment and continue to grow. Tubes with TSB with NaCl (6.5%) are inoculated with a bacterial sample and incubated at 37 °C. A positive finding occurs if the solution becomes cloudy from the growth of organisms.

Mannitol salt agar test contains mannitol (10 g), a sugar; beef extract (1 g); proteose peptone #3 (10 g); NaCl 75 g, agar (15 g), phenol red (0.025 g), a pH indicator; and 1 distilled water (1000 mL). The solution is heated until clear, autoclaved at 121 °C, cooled and poured into Petri dishes. The high salt concentration inhibits most bacteria, but *Staphylococcus* species are able to ferment the mannitol, and this produces an acid that changes the pH of the phenol and causes the agar to change from red to yellow.

Bacitracin disks contain 0.04 units of bacitracin, to which group A *Streptococcus* is susceptible. The disk is placed on top of a blood agar plate covering zone one (area that is heavily inoculated with a specimen) and incubated. If growth is inhibited about the disk, this is an indication of group A *Streptococcus.*

Bile solubility test is done to identify *S. pneumoniae.* A drop of 10% sodium deoxycholate is placed on top of an established suspected colony (after 18–24 hours of growth) and then incubated for 15–30 minutes at 37 °C. If *S. pneumoniae* is present, this procedure will cause lysis of the cells.

Coagulase bile esculin (*Enterococcus* slant) test is done to identify *Enterococcus.* The medium contains beef extract (3 g), peptone (5 g), oxgall (40 g), esculin (0.5 g), ferric citrate (0.5 g), agar (15 g), and distilled water (1000 mL). The solution is heated, pH adjust to 7.09, autoclaved at 121 °C for 15 minutes, cooled to 55 °C, and poured into sterile tubes and allowed to set with the tubes in slanted rather than upright position. (Note: Before filling tubes, 50 mL horse serum may be added to the solution, but this is optional). Once the agar has set, inoculate the slants with organisms from the primary plate. *Enterococcus,* which is esculin positive, will form brown-black colonies with a surrounding black zone.

NAGLER TEST

The Nagler test is used to identify bacterial organisms that can produce lecithinases (phospholipases). One example of such an organism is *Clostridium perfringens.* Place the sample in question on an agar medium containing egg yolk. On one half of the agar medium, add the antitoxin for *Clostridium perfringens* type A. After incubation, a positive Nagler test will show the half of the test plate that contains the antitoxin is clear and has no evidence of lecithinase production. The half of the test plate that did not contain the antitoxin will show evidence of the production of lecithinase as an opaque area surrounding the bacterial sample.

NIACIN TEST

The niacin test is used to identify the presence of a specific type of mycobacteria, *Mycobacterium tuberculosis.* This particular mycobacterium releases a large quantity of niacin (B$_3$) during its metabolic processes. All mycobacteria release a certain amount of niacin, but only Mycobacterium tuberculosis releases enough to be of use in the niacin test. Culture the sample on egg based media for a three to four week incubation period before niacin testing. Add a cyanogen bromide (CNBr) solution and an aniline solution to the egg based bacterial culture. If niacin is present, a color change to yellow will be seen. If there is no color change, then *Mycobacterium tuberculosis* is not present. Care should be taken when performing the niacin test because cyanogen bromide solution is highly toxic. Wear a respirator, gloves, and use a fume hood.

ISOLATING, IDENTIFYING, AND DIFFERENTIATING BACTERIA
GRAM-POSITIVE COCCI

When gram-staining, gram-positive organisms stain purple and gram-negative organisms stain red ("Purple for positive"). Hemolysis may occur as a reaction on blood agar plates: Alpha (hemoglobin converts to form that appears shows as green, Beta (true hemolysis), and Gamma (nonhemoloytic).

Gram-positive cocci include:

Genera	Species	Differentiation
Staphylococcus (catalase positive and occur in clusters)	S. aureus	Beta/gamma hemolytic, positive for coagulase positive for mannitol fermentation, sensitive to novobiocin.
	S. epidermidis	Gamma hemolytic, negative for coagulase production, negative for mannitol fermentation, sensitive to novobiocin.
	S. saprophyticus	Same as *S. epidermidis* except resistant to novobiocin.
Streptococcus (catalase negative, grow in chains)	S. pyogenes	Lancefield group A, Beta hemolytic, sensitive to bacitracin (A disc).
	S. agalactiae	Lancefield group B, Beta or gamma hemolytic, positive CAMP tests
	S. pneumoniae	Non-groupable, Alpha hemolytic, bile soluble, sensitive to optochin (P disc).
Enterococcus	E. faecalis	Lancefield group D, Gamma hemolytic. Ferments mannitol and grows on mannitol salt agar

Genera	Species	Differentiation
(catalase negative, similar to strep)	E. faecium.	Lancefield group D, Gamma hemolytic. Does not ferment mannitol or grow on mannitol salt agar.

GRAM-POSITIVE BACILLI

Genera	Species	Differentiation
Bacillus (spore producing)	B. anthracis	Associated with anthrax infection.
		Large cell, end-to-end chains, no motility, has poly-D-glutamic acid capsule.
	B. cereus	Associated with GI infections.
		Large cell, 50% of strains are motile.
Corynebacterium	C. diphtheriae	Associated with diphtheria.
		Small, narrow cell, no spores, no motility, pleomorphic, Chinese characters.
Listeria	L. monocytogenes	Associated with listeriosis, GI infection.
		Small cell. No spores, motility (tumbling), grow at 4°C intracellularly.

GRAM-NEGATIVE COCCI

Genera	Species	Differentiation
Neisseria (Diplococci)	N. gonorrhoeae	Associated with sexually-transmitted disease.
		Positive oxidase, coffee-bean shaped, glucose positive, maltose negative, media—chocolate and Thayer-Martin agar.
	N. meningitidis	Associated with meningitis.
		Positive oxidase, kidney-bean shaped, glucose positive, maltose positive, media—blood or chocolate agar.
Moraxella (Diplococcus)	M. catarrhalis	Associated with respiratory infection.
		Positive oxidase, kidney-bean shaped, glucose negative, maltose negative, media—blood or chocolate agar.

GRAM-NEGATIVE COCCOBACILLI

Genera	Species	Differentiation
Haemophilus (influenza)	H. influenzae	Needs both factor X (hemin) and V (NAD) to grow. Cannot grow on blood agar but will grow about a streak line of β-hemolytic Staphylococcus aureus on blood agar (satellitism) because the Staph liberates factor. Media—Chocolate agar
	H. ducreyi	Needs only factor X to grow Media—Chocolate agar and rabbit blood agar
Acinetobacter (HA infections)	A. baumannii	Standard ID not available. Differentiated by multiplex PCR OXA-51 typing.
Kingella (Invasive infections)	K. Kingae	In pairs or chains, often resistive to gram staining, beta-hemolytic, nonmotile, does not form spores. Negative catalase, negative urease, and negative indol tests but usually positive to oxidase.
Francisella (Tularemia)	F. tularensis	Non-motile, does not form spores Media—Chocolate agar (enriched), buffered charcoal yeast extract Culture often not successful, so ID is by DNA methods, immunoblotting, and antigen ELISA.

GRAM-NEGATIVE BACILLI (RODS)

Genera	Species	Differentiation
Bacteroides	*B. fragilis*	Rod-shaped, non-motile, negative oxidase, Negative H_2S gas, obligate anaerobic.
Campylobacter	*C. jejuni*	Comma, corkscrew, or S-shaped, motile, negative glucose fermentation, positive oxidase, negative lactose fermentation, negative H_2S gas, and growth optimal at 42 °C. Microaerophilic.
	C. coli	S-shaped. Similar to *C. jejuni*. Differentiated from *C. jejuni* by real-time assay.
	C. fetus	S-shaped, motile, microaerophilic, growth optimal on Butzler agar and CCDA agar, but no growth on MacConkey agar, catalase and oxidase positive, colistin-resistant.
Escherichia	*E. coli*	Rod-shaped, motile, positive glucose fermentation, negative oxidase, positive lactose fermentation, and negative H_2S gas.
Helicobacter	*H. pylori*	Spiral-shaped, motile, negative glucose fermentation, positive oxidase, negative lactose fermentation, and negative H_2S gas. Produces urease.
Salmonella	*S. enterica*	Rod-shaped, motile, positive glucose fermentation, Negative oxidase, negative lactose fermentation, and positive H_2S gas. Black on hektoen agar.
	S. typhi	Rod-shaped, facultative anaerobe, has H, O, and Vi antigens, catalase positive, oxidase and urease negative, vancomycin resistant, colistin susceptible. Black on hektoen agar.
Shigella	*S. flexneri*	Rod-shaped, nonmotile, positive glucose fermentation, negative oxidase, negative lactose fermentation, negative H_2S gas.
	S. dysenteriae	Rod-shaped, non-spore forming, facultative anaerobe, nonmotile, negative lactose fermentation and negative lysine. Green on hektoen agar.
Yersinia	*Y. enterocolitica*	Rod-shaped, nonmotile, positive glucose fermentation, negative oxidase, negative lactose fermentation, and negative H_2S gas.
Vibrio	*V. parahaemolyticus*	Comma-shaped, motile, facultative anaerobe, non-spore forming, positive glucose fermentation, positive glucose fermentation, negative lactose fermentation, negative H_2S gas. Optimal growth in high salt environment.
	V. vulnificus	Facultative anaerobe, non-spore forming, motile, curved or straight rods. Negative growth in 0% NaCl and positive in 1% NaCl. Positive lactose fermentation, positive oxidase, positive nitrate to nitrite, negative myo-inositol fermentation, negative arginine dihydrolase, positive lysine decarboxylase, 10–89% positive ornithine decarboxylase.

69

Genera	Species	Differentiation
	V. cholerae	Facultative anaerobe, non-spore forming, motile, positive growth in 0% and 1% NaCl, negative lactose fermentation, oxidase positive, positive nitrate to nitrite, negative myo-inositol fermentation, negative arginine dihydrolase, positive lysine decarboxylase and ornithine decarboxylase.

ENTEROBACTERIACEAE

Bacteria belonging to the family Enterobacteriaceae are gram-negative, anerobic, rod-shaped bacteria. They also produce lactic acid by fermenting sugars. Most of the Enterobacteriaceae are mobile, using flagella to move, but a few members are non-mobile. Bacteria from this family are normal flora in the guts and intestines of healthy humans, in soil or water, or in plants. Some are parasitic. Some examples of bacteria that belong to the family Enterobacteriaceae are *E. coli* and *Salmonella*.

USING TRIPLE SUGAR IRON AGAR (TSI) TEST IN ENTERIC IDENTIFICATION

Laboratory technicians often use the triple sugar iron agar test to differentiate among various kinds of *Enterobacteriaceae* bacteria. This is an especially useful test, because it can give data on glucose fermentation, lactose fermentation, sucrose fermentation and H_2S formation. There are four possible results for a TSI test:

- Yellow (acid) deep: yellow bacteria, glucose positive
- Yellow slant (acid): light yellow bacteria, sucrose or lactose positive
- Alkaline slant/alkaline deep: bacteria are not members of *Enterobacteriaceae*, since they are not fermenters
- Alkaline slant/acid deep: red or yellow bacteria, glucose positive and non-lactose fermenters

MRSA AND ITS IMPORTANCE IN HEALTHCARE-ASSOCIATED INFECTIONS (HAIS)

Methicillin-resistant *Staphylococcus aureus* (MRSA) was first identified in 1961 in Europe after the development and overuse of synthetic penicillins caused *Staphylococcus aureus* to mutate into resistant strains. Since 1961, MRSA has infected millions of people worldwide. MRSA is resistant to methicillin and other β-lactam antibiotics, such as amoxicillin and oxacillin, and sometimes other classes of antibiotics. *Staphylococcus* is able to form biofilms, which aids in resistance. **Healthcare-associated MRSA infections** most commonly involve surgical sites, urinary tract, blood stream, and lungs (pneumonia). Because of increased awareness and better practices, MRSA HAIs decreased by 54% between 2004 and 2011 but still pose a threat to patients because of the severity of some infections and the risk of resistance to other drugs. **Community-acquired MRSA** most commonly results in skin infections, such as folliculitis, and can easily spread to others where groups of people are in close contact, such as in day cares, gyms, schools, and barracks.

MULTI-DRUG-RESISTANT ORGANISMS

MDROs are those that have mutated and developed forms that are resistant to multiple antibiotics. Initially, resistance developed to one class of antibiotics, such as β-lactams, which resulted in methicillin-resistant *Staphylococcus aureus* infections and penicillin-resistant *Streptococcus pneumoniae,* but bacteria continued to mutate, becoming resistant to more classes of antibiotics and severely limiting the antibiotic arsenal needed for treatment. Of current concern is extended-spectrum beta-lactamases (ESBLs), resistant to cephalosporins and monobactams; and multi-drug-resistant tuberculosis (MDR).

VANCOMYCIN-RESISTANT *ENTEROCOCCUS*

Up until the 1980s, most enterococci responded to vancomycin, a strong antibiotic, but the increased use of antibiotics for all types of infection resulted in mutations that rendered some enterococci species vancomycin-resistant (VRE), leaving few options for treatment of severe infection. There are currently 6 different forms (A-G) of vancomycin resistance. For example, the Van-A form is resistant to vancomycin and teicoplanin (an alternative antibiotic for severe infections).

Special Tests

STREPTOCOCCAL TESTING

Streptococcus infections include strep throat, scarlet fever, rheumatic fever, necrotizing fasciitis, urinary tract infections, psoriasis, and pneumonia.

Throat swabs: rapid enzyme immunoassay (more accurate for positives than negatives) (group A)	A number of different rapid strep kits are available that are able to detect strep group A. The tests usually begin with a tonsillar and throat swab. The swab is then swirled inside of a tube holding a mixture of 2 reagents, left in place for about 1 minute, and then removed and a test strip inserted, timed, and checked against a color chart. Antibody/antigen sensitivity tests also help to identify strep.
Beta-hemolytic strep (group B) screening for *S. agalactiae*.	Commonly colonizes in intestinal, urinary, and reproductive systems and can infect the fetus in late pregnancy, so screening of pregnant women is done routinely with rectal and vaginal cultures because most are asymptomatic. While the strep is not usually pathogenic to the mother, the newborn may develop pneumonia (newborns lack alveolar macrophages) or meningitis.
Bacterial identification	Streptococci are gram-positive cocci that occur in pairs or chains and are facultative anaerobes. Streptococci grow on blood agar, chocolate agar, and (some species) on PEA. Cultured colonies are small, gray, and slightly raised and appear translucent with a margin around the entire colony.
	Streptococci are catalase negative, esculin negative, MSA, and optochin negative, and these tests can differentiate strep from other cocci.
	Alpha-hemolytic strep (*S. pneumoniae*, which is optochin susceptible and bile soluble) exhibits only partial hemolysis.
	Beta-hemolytic strep includes group A strep (*S. pyogenes*, which exhibit strong beta-hemolysis and bacitracin inhibition) and group B strep (*S. agalactiae*, identified by the CAMP test). Beta-hemolytic strep cases complete hemolysis.

CLOSTRIDIUM DIFFICILE TOXIN TESTS

Clostridium difficile can release a toxin that can cause necrosis of the colon. A variety of tests are available to test stool for ***Clostridium difficile* toxin**, and the time needed may vary from a few hours to several days (more sensitive). The two-step procedure is recommended:

- Step 1: Glutamate dehydrogenase (GDH) test: This is a rapid screening test that shows if the *Clostridium difficile*-produced antigen, glutamate dehydrogenase, is present, but does not differentiate between strains that produce toxin and those that do not.

- Step 2 choices:
  - Cell cytotoxicity culture (takes 24-48 hours): Tissue test that identifies the cytotoxin on tissue cells.
  - Stool culture on fresh stool (takes 2-3 days): Can identify toxin but not cannot differentiate colonization from overgrowth of the organism, so further toxin testing, such as tests for toxin A and B, must be done. Testing should be done as soon as possible or sample refrigerated as toxins rapidly degrade.
  - PCR assay: Results are available rapidly and test is sensitive but is expensive and not widely available.

CAMPYLOBACTER PYLORI SCREENING

Microscopic	Microorganism may be observed in the feces in a fresh specimen (≤2 hours) or from cultures.
Culture & Sensitivities	Microorganism is more difficult than other enteric microorganism to culture and requires use of special blood agar that contains antibiotics, micropore filtration, and incubation at 42 °C.
ELISA	Antigen testing allows for serodiagnosis.
PCR	Able to directly detect the microorganism in stool.
Serology	Tests for presence of antibodies, but they may not be detected early in the infection so the test should be repeated within 10–14 days.
Rapid urease (RUT)	6% RUT most accurate and test results may be available within 10 minutes (compared to other microorganisms that show positive results after a longer period of time).

HELICOBACTER PYLORI SCREENING

Antigen	Fecal test often used for diagnosis. Positive if the *H. pylori* antigen or traces of the microorganism are detected.
Antibody	Serum test can identify antibodies to *H. pylori* but cannot differentiate previous infection from current, so not used for diagnosis and positive finding must be confirmed.
Urea breath	Solution containing urea is swallowed and level of carbon dioxide measured in exhaled breaths 10 minutes later as H. pylori converts urea to carbon dioxide.
Microscopic	Tissue sample (GI) may show presence of *H. pylori*.
Culture & sensitivities	Culture of *H. pylori* is generally done only if necessary susceptibility testing for antibiotics.
Rapid urease	The enzyme urease (produced by *H. pylori)* may be detected in tissue sample.
PCR	Generally not necessary for diagnosis but may be used for research purposes.

SHIGA TOXIN TESTS

Shiga toxin tests are used to isolate and confirm the presence of microorganisms that produce Shiga toxins. A fresh stool specimen should be collected in 3-tube stool kit as soon as possible after onset of diarrhea and prior to beginning antibiotic therapy. The specimen may be maintained at room temperature for 24 hours and under refrigeration for 2 days. The screening may be done through PCR, EIA, or culture. Shiga testing kits, such as BioStar® OIA SHIGATOX test, are available commercially to help identify strains. Identification of some strains of Shiga toxin–producing microorganisms may require sending the sample to a state public health laboratory. For example, some strains of *E. coli* are Shiga-producing, and stool cultures are not able to detect all strains, so EIAs, which are not always readily available because of cost, are required for testing.

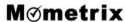

ANTIMICROBIAL SUSCEPTIBILITY TESTING

Antimicrobial susceptibility testing is done to determine which antibiotic an organism is susceptible to. The Kirby-Bauer test (disk diffusion test) is one method:

- Select 3 to 5 colonies and prepare with direct colony suspension or the log phase method.
- Inoculate a Mueller-Hinton agar plate (4 mm depth) or other medium specific to the organism.
- Apply antimicrobial disks individually or with automatic disk dispenser within 15 minutes of inoculation.
- Invert plate and incubate at required temperature and duration, generally between 16 and 24 hours.
- Measures zones of inhibition from the back of the plate, using reflected or transmitted light depending on the organism.

Many factors can affect the results of manual testing: incubation temperature and duration, type of medium, bacterial growth rate, depth of the medium, procedures for reading results. Automated systems generally provide more reliable results and have test panels available for specific organisms as well as gram-positive and gram-negative bacteria.

MINIMUM INHIBITORY CONCENTRATION (MIC) TESTING

Minimum inhibitory concentration (MIC) testing is used to determine the lowest antimicrobial concentration that is effective in inhibiting growth of the organism. Commercial plates and panels are available. For example, the broth microdilution MIC test includes a panel with 96 wells (0.1 mL) for inoculation while the agar dilution MIC test includes agar medium plates with different antimicrobial concentrations; however, the MIC test with agar plates is time consuming and more difficult to quantify. Incubation duration varies from 16–24 hours, depending on the organism. The MIC endpoint is the concentration at which growth is completely inhibited or >80% compared to the control for some antibiotics. Automated systems are available for antimicrobial susceptibility testing. For example, a well card may be automatically incubated and read by a photometer and the MIC calculated by a computerized program.

FECAL OCCULT BLOOD AND IMMUNOCHEMICAL TESTS

Stool may be examined macroscopically for volume, odor, color, consistency, mucus, and microscopically to identify the presence of cells (leukocytes, epithelial cells) and other materials (meat fibers). **Tests for occult blood** commonly include:

- **Fecal occult blood test (FOBT):** This test detects blood that has occurred from anywhere in the digestive tract because the blood reacts to the guaiac the test card is coated with. This test cannot distinguish between bleeding from the upper GI tract and the lower GI tract, so it is less specific than the FIT.
- **Fecal immunochemical test (FIT):** This test detects blood in the stool from lower GI bleeding through the use of antibodies against human hemoglobin (so it does not react to animal hemoglobin from ingested meats). FIT does not detect upper GI bleeding because the hemoglobin has been broken down by the digestive process by the time it reaches the rectum and is expelled.

MOLECULAR ASSAYS IN BACTERIOLOGY

Molecular assays in bacteriology are able to identify bacteria or specific strains of bacteria based on their genetic sequences. Test results are usually available within hours rather than the days that may be required for cultures. A number of different tests are available:

- Direct PCR/gene sequencing: Sterile body fluid/tissue specimen used for amplification and sequencing. Isolates identified by sequencing of ribosomal RNA (purified DNA not necessary).
- Direct real time PCR for specific pathogens: Mycobacterium tuberculosis, Clostridium difficile, Bordetella pertussis, Bordetella parapertussis, Shiga-toxin producing Escherichia coli (including serotypes), Salmonella enterica, Shigella spp., group B Streptococcus agalactiae, Streptococcus pyogenes, and Streptococcus group C/G.
- PCR gene detection: MecA and BlaZ.
- Pulsed field gel electrophoresis strain typing: Used to identify different strains of organisms, such as *Staphylococcus aureus.*
- Multiplex PCR: Multiple targets are amplified in one PCR test.

Virology

BLOT TESTS

The **Western blot test** is used in the laboratory to help confirm or deny the presence of HIV virus. Unlike the Southern blot and Northern blot tests, this test can test for both DNA and RNA protein fragments. Gel electrophoresis is used to separate these fragments of the viruses' DNA and RNA, and then they are covered with a membrane composed of nitrocellulose. The patient's serum is reacted with these separated DNA and RNA fragments. If the patient's serum contains antibodies for the HIV virus, those antibodies will bind to the DNA and RNA fragments present. This binding will produce a characteristic pattern (referred to as the characteristic blot), which can then be visualized. This pattern can then confirm the presence of the HIV virus in the patient's blood serum.

The **Southern blot test** is used to identify DNA (deoxyribonucleic acid) fragments in the laboratory. In this test, gel electrophoresis is used to separate fragments of DNA. Then, these fragments are covered with a membrane consisting of nitrocellulose. Finally, a specific probe is used to identify the fragments of DNA.

The **Northern blot test** is used to identify RNA (ribonucleic acid) sequences in the laboratory. First, fragments of RNA are separated using gel electrophoresis. Then, as in the Southern blot test, the fragments are covered with a nitrocellulose membrane. Lastly, a specific probe for this procedure is used to identify the RNA sequences present.

MEASLES

The measles is a virus that most often affects children of school age, and most often children in developing countries. In the United States, vaccination against the measles in early childhood is recommended. The measles is easily spread from human to human, and it enters the body through the respiratory system by inhalation. The virus multiplies in the respiratory system, and spreads through the circulatory system. Some of the symptoms of the measles are: A characteristic body rash that appears within 14 days of being infected, a high fever, red eyes, sneezing, and cough. Also, Koplik's spots may be seen. These spots are small and reddish with a bluish-white spot in their centers, and appear in the mouth, but since they only persist for a short time, their presence may not be noted. Complications, such as pneumonia, can arise from the measles. The presence of measles IgM antibodies can be detected through serum analysis. Most cases of the measles last about seven to ten days.

TYPES OF SAMPLES TO TEST FOR GASTROENTERITIS, ENCEPHALITIS, VIRAL MENINGITIS, AND CUTANEOUS RASHES

Condition	Sample Type	Possible Cause
Gastroenteritis	Stool samples or rectal swabs	Adenovirus or calicivirus
Encephalitis	Brain biopsy or serum sample	Herpes simplex virus one (HSV-1), arbovirus, or varicella-zoster virus (VZV)
Viral meningitis	Urine samples, serum samples, stool samples, throat swabs, or cerebral spinal fluid samples	VZV, herpes simplex virus two (HSV-2), enterovirus, mumps, or lymphocytic choriomeningitis virus
Cutaneous rashes	Throat swabs, urine samples, stool samples, or serum samples	HSV-1, HSV-2, measles, rubella, Epstein-Barr virus, parvovirus B-19, enterovirus, echovirus, and cytomegalovirus

CHICKENPOX VS. SHINGLES

Both chickenpox and shingles are caused by the varicella-zoster virus, which is a kind of herpesvirus 90 to 100 nanometers large. These viruses are icosahedral in shape and contain DNA. Shingles mainly occurs in adult humans and is considered to be a reactivation of the chickenpox virus that takes place in the peripheral or cranial nerves. Symptoms include pain and skin vesicles, which, if left untreated, can deteriorate into eye problems and central nervous system disorders. Chickenpox typically affects children, and has a characteristic rash as its main symptom. Chickenpox is usually spread by means of airborne droplets.

SIZE AND SHAPE OF ORTHOMYXOVIRUS, PARAMYXOVIRUS, RETROVIRUS, RHABDOVIRUS, REOVIRUS, AND HERPESVIRUS

Virus	Size (nm)	Contents	Shape	Example
Orthomyxovirus	75–125	RNA	Helical	Influenza
Paramyxovirus	150–300	RNA	Helical	Mumps
Retrovirus	80–130	RNA	Icosahedral	HIV
Rhabdovirus	150–350	RNA	Bullet	Rabies
Reovirus	50–80	RNA	Icosahedral	Rotavirus
Herpes virus	90–100	DNA	Icosahedral	Herpes simplex virus

HEPATITIS A VIRUS AND HEPATITIS B VIRUS

	Hepatitis A virus (HAV)	Hepatitis B virus (HBV)
Size	24–30 nm	42–47 nm
Contents	RNA with no envelope	DNA, Dane particles, and an envelope
Shape	Icosahedral	Spherical
Effects	Nausea, jaundice, and anorexia	Liver failure
Incubation	15–40 days	50–80 days
Route	Fecal to oral, typically because of poor food sanitation practices	Contaminated body fluids, often during tattoos, needle sticks, and intravenous drug use
Notes	Low mortality rate	Vaccines have been developed

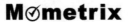

Parasitology

HELMINTHS

Helminths are parasitic worms that live in humans, primarily in the intestines. There are a variety of helminths, including roundworms, tapeworms, pinworms, flukes, and the worm *Trichinella spiralis*, which is responsible for causing trichinosis. Eggs from helminths can contaminate a variety of things, including feces, pets and other animals, water, air, food, and surfaces like toilet seats. Eggs of helminths usually enter a human via the anus, the nose, or the mouth, and they then travel to the intestines, where they hatch, grow, and multiply. The presence of helminths can be determined in most cases by examining stool samples of suspected infected individuals. Drugs known as vermifuges can be used to treat infections from helminth worms. To prevent infection from helminths, thoroughly cook meats, keep a clean kitchen and bathroom, and wash hands frequently.

SPECIMENS AND PRESERVATION METHODS FOR PARASITOLOGY TESTING

Stool is the most common parasite specimen collected. Samples must be collected into a clean, dry container with a secure lid, and they must not be contaminated by urine, water, or enemas. Contamination from urine has the ability to destroy motile organisms, water may contain free living organisms, and protozoa may not be detectable for 5 to 10 days following the administration of barium enemas. Recovery of parasites may be hindered up to 2 weeks after the cessation of certain antibiotics. The most concentrated, early morning and first-void **sputum** and **urine** specimens are collected into dry, sterile containers with a secure lid. **Genital swabs** submitted for parasitic detection require saline to keep them moist for optimal organism recovery. **Skin** and **tissue** samples are best submitted to the laboratory in dry, sterile containers with a secure lid. Fresh **blood** from a fingerstick is the preferred sample for thick and thin blood smear preparations; however, blood collection via venipuncture into an EDTA tube is also acceptable.

Methods of sample storage and preservation based on the type of parasite suspected are as follows:

- **Refrigeration:** eggs, larvae, and amoebic cysts. If amoebic trophozoites are suspected, do not refrigerate.
- 10% formalin and merthiolate-iodine-formalin: eggs, larvae, and amoebic cysts.
- **Polyvinyl alcohol (PVA):** amoebic trophozoites; stained specimen slides can be permanently preserved using this method.
- **Sodium acetate-acetic acid-formalin:** amoebic trophozoites; an environmentally safer alternative to PVA.
- **Schaudinn's fluid:** trophs and cysts, fixative for fresh stool samples.

MACROSCOPIC IDENTIFICATION

Ova, cyst, and parasite examinations begin with the evaluation of macroscopic properties of the sample. Characteristics including the consistency, color, and presence of certain substances indicate the presence of a parasitic infection and provide information toward obtaining a positive parasite identification.

The **consistency** of a stool specimen can indicate which form of a parasite will exist in the specimen. Helminth eggs may be present in stool of any consistency, whereas formed stools contain protozoan cysts, soft stools contain trophozoites or cysts, and liquid stool samples will contain trophozoites. Stool can be macroscopically examined for the presence of **mucus, blood,** or **macroscopic parasites.** The **color** of stool samples can also provide insight to the presence of parasitic infections. Black stools indicate the presence of iron or blood, and light-tan or white stool

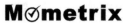

samples indicate barium or the absence of bile, all of which indicate the presence of parasites in the gastrointestinal tract.

MICROSCOPIC OBSERVATION AND IDENTIFICATION OF PARASITES

Ova and parasites are identified microscopically by key characteristics using a variety of stains and slide preparations. Fresh samples can be observed as a **wet mount**, mixed with saline to observe motility and iodine to kill trophozoites and enhance nuclear material. Fresh and preserved specimens can be permanently stained for the detection, identification, quantification, and permanent recording of parasites. The **trichrome** stain is the most common stain used for identifying intestinal parasites. It is rapid and simple, and it yields uniformly stained parasites, yeast, human cells, and artifacts. Cysts, trophozoites, and small protozoa undetected on wet mount can be identified with trichrome stains. The **modified trichrome** stain is diagnostic for detecting unicellular, intracellular microsporidian parasites. Blood smears stained with **Wright** and **Giemsa** stains provide rapid detection of malarial parasite rings in RBCs. **Acid-fast** staining identifies coccidian oocysts that are difficult to detect with other stains, and it is diagnostic for *Cryptosporidium, Isospora*, and *Cyclospora* species. Intestinal parasites can be quantified and their microfilarial sheath can be observed by staining with **iron hematoxylin**.

Key microscopic characteristics evaluated for helminth eggs and other parasite identification include:

- **Shape**: oval, round, ellipse, symmetrical, elongated, lightbulb or barrel shaped
- **Size**: measured in microns
- **Color:** colorless, yellow, brown
- **Texture, outer shell appearance:** operculated, smooth, scalloped edge, lateral or terminal spine, polar or bipolar filaments.

If recovered, adult worms can be observed for key identifying features including flat or round body shape, pointed or notched tails, the shape and number of teeth, sheath, and the presence and arrangement of nuclei on the tail.

TYPES, CLASSIFICATIONS, DESCRIPTION, AND IDENTIFICATION OF PARASITES IN CLINICAL SPECIMENS
PARASITES: PROTISTS (PROTOZOA—ONE-CELLED ANIMAL FORM)

Type and Classification	Description	Identification
Intestinal flagellates: *Giardia lamblia, Trichomonas vaginalis, Dientamoeba fragilis* **Hemoflagellates**: *Trypanosoma, Leishmania, Trypanosoma cruzi*	Contain one or more flagella (whip-like tails), and some have undulating membrane.	Identify cysts or trophozoites in fecal smears, PCR, EIA, antigen detection.
Intestinal amoebas: *Entamoeba histolytica, Balantidium coli*	Stages: amoeba, inactive cyst, and intermediate precyst. Move with pseudopodia.	Identify cysts in stool specimen, EIA, antigen detection, PCR.
Blood apicomplexa/ sporozoa: *Plasmodium vivax, ovale, malariae*, and *falciparum*; *Isospora belli; Babesia microti, sarcocystis* spp.; *Cryptosporidium* spp; *Toxoplasma gondii*	Spore-forming with organelle to penetrate host cell.	Plasmodium: Thick and thin Giemsa-stained blood film to identify organisms, antigen-capture tests. Others: Identify oocysts in fresh stool, PCR, EIA, DFA, GPP.

77

Type and Classification	Description	Identification
Microsporida: *Encephalitozoon hellum, Enterocytozoon bieneusi, encephalitozoon intestinalis*	One-celled spore with tubular polar filament to inject sporoplasm into host where it develops.	Electron microscopy to identify spore, nuclei, and polar filament.
Ciliates: *Balantidium coli*	Organism with cilia in rows/patches and 2 kinds of nuclei.	Identifying cysts or trophozoites in stool.

Helminths (Parasitic Worms)

Type and Classification	Description	Identification
Nematoda (Round worms): *Ascaris lumbricoides, Anisakis* spp. (cod/herring worms), *Enterobius vermicularis* (pinworms), *Strongyloides stercoralis, Ancylostoma duodenale/Necator americanus* (hookworm)	Size varies from 0.3 mm to 8 m, long, narrow non-segmented cylindrical body. Stages include egg, larva filariform and/or rhabditiform, and adult.	Identify eggs, parasites, or larvae in stool specimen. Pinworms: Cellophane tape test.
Cestoda (Tapeworms): *Hymenolepis nana* (dwarf tapeworm), *Taenia saginata* (beef tapeworm, *Taenia solium* (pork tapeworm), *Diphyllobothrium latum* (fish tapeworm)	Long, flat, segmented worms with scolex (head/sucker), neck, and strobila (segments). Stages include egg/gravid proglottids, oncosphere, cysticercus, cysticercoid, and adult.	Identify proglottids and eggs or scolex in stool specimen.
Trematoda (flatworms/flukes): *Fasciolopsis buski, Heterophyes, Schistosoma* spp.	Flat, leaf-shaped, non-segmented worms. Stages may include egg, miracidium, sporocyst, redia, cercariae, metacercariae, excyst, and adult.	Identify eggs in stool specimen.

Trichrome Stain

The trichrome stain is a permanent stain that allows for visualization of and morphological distinguishing of parasitic cysts and trophozoites in clinical specimens. The most common specimens submitted for trichrome staining are fresh or preserved stool fecal samples; however, other clinical specimens are able to be stained with polyvinyl alcohol (PVA) fixation.

The trichrome stain consists of chromotrope 2R, light green SF, phosphotungstic acid, glacial acetic acid, and distilled water. Stain preparation is necessary, by adding 1 ml of acetic acid to the dry components, allowing the mixture to stand for 30 minutes, and then adding 100 ml of distilled water. The stain should be purple in color and should be protected from light. Proper fixation of slides is included in the trichrome procedure because it is necessary for quality staining and optimal use of this method.

Trichrome procedure:

1. Prepare a fresh fecal smear or PVA smear.
2. Place the slide in 70% ETOH for 5 minutes — for PVA smears, skip this step.
3. Remove the slide and drain off the excess liquid.

4. Place the slide in 70% ETOH with added iodine (dark reddish-brown color) for 2 to 5 minutes.
5. Remove the slide and drain off the excess liquid.
6. Place the slide in 70% ETOH for 5 minutes.
7. Remove the slide and drain off the excess liquid.
8. Place the slide in clean/new 70% ETOH for 2 to 5 minutes.
9. Remove the slide and drain off the excess liquid.
10. Place the slide in a prepared trichrome stain solution for 10 minutes.
11. Remove the slide and drain off the excess stain.
12. Dip the slide in 90% ETOH acidified with 1% acetic acid up to 3 seconds (no longer).
13. Dip once in 100% ETOH.
14. Place the slide in 100% ETOH for 2 to 5 minutes.
15. Place the slide in clean/new 100% ETOH for 2 to 5 minutes.
16. Place the slide in xylene for 2 to 5 minutes.
17. Repeat the slide in xylene for 2 to 5 minutes.
18. Mount the slide with a cover glass, and allow it to dry overnight at 37 °C.
19. Observe with a fluorescent microscope.

Outcome:

- Background debris — green
- Protozoa — blue-green to purple; the nuclei and inclusions of parasites will show red to purple-red.

Mycology

MYCOLOGICAL ORGANISMS (FUNGI)

Most fungi are aerobic and have at least 1 nucleus. Fungi secrete enzymes and are part of natural microbial flora. Yeasts: Single cell spherical/ellipsoid 3-15 μm in diameter. Some produce buds and chains of buds called pseudohyphae. Colonies are 1-3 mm in size, cream colored. Molds: Growth is per multicellular filamentous colonies with branching intertwined tubules called hyphae, which are 2-10 μm in diameter. Fungi may be classified in a number of ways, but for medical purposes classification according to the site of infection is most common. Fungi are often described by appearance as cottony, powdery, velvety, or glabrous (waxy).

Classification	Types	Description
Superficial mycoses	Pityriasis versicolor (*Malassezia* spp, tinea nigra, piedra)	Invade superficial layers of skin and hair shaft.
Cutaneous mycoses	Tinea corporis, tinea pedis, tinea cruris, tinea capitis, tinea barbae, tinea unguium, dermatophytid	Infect superficial keratinized tissue, such as hair, skin, and nails. Unable to grow if serum is present or temperature is ≥37 °C.
Subcutaneous mycoses	*Sporothrix schenckii,* chromoblastomycosis, phaeohyphomycosis, mycetoma, *Coccidioides immitis, Coccidioides posadasii*	Normally grow in soil or vegetation and infect through traumatic inoculation. Infections are usually subcutaneous but in rare cases spread systemically.

79

Classification	Types	Description
Endemic mycoses	Coccidioidomycosis, histoplasmosis, blastomycosis, paracoccidioidomycosis, candidiasis, aspergillosis, sporotrichosis	Most infections result from inhalation in immunocompromised individuals. Infections cause inflammatory response and production of cell-mediated immunity and antibodies.

MYCOLOGICAL PROCEDURES TO IDENTIFY FUNGI

Exoantigen test	The exoantigen test is a gel immunodiffusion precipitin test in which soluble antigens produced by fungi grown in broth media react with anti-serum (produced from rabbits injected with antigens), allowing for identification of dimorphic fungi. Fungi are identified according the presence of specific antigens. This test has been generally supplanted by DNA probe testing.
DNA probe	DNA probe testing is more efficient and less time-consuming than the exoantigen test and poses les risk to laboratory workers. A DNA probe is a DNA fragment that is labeled with a fluorescent or radioactive material and can recognize genes in DNA sequences of specific organisms. Procedures vary widely, depending upon the specific type of test, but PCR probe-based tests are available for mycological studies to identify pathogenic fungi.

DERMATOPHYTES

Dermatophytes are a type of pathogenic and parasitic fungi. These fungi most often cause infections of skin, hair, and nails, on humans and other animals. Two types of infections caused by dermatophytes are tinea and ringworm. There are three genera of dermatophytes: *Epidermophyton*, *Microsporum*, and *Trichophyton*. In the laboratory, they can be identified on Sabouraud's agar. Examination of the morphology of the macroconidia and the microconidia produced is a very reliable method for identification of dermatophytes. Sometimes, stimulating spore production in the sample can also be useful in dermatophyte identification. However, coloring and texture of the fungi can be variable, so these characteristics are not very reliable in dermatophyte identification.

FUNGAL PATHOGENS

Most fungal species are often first identified by Gram stain procedures or microscopic examination of urine sediment. In a Gram stain, yeast will appear as budding cells or pseudohyphae pigmented purple or a blue-black color. Preparing hair, skin, or nail samples with potassium hydroxide (KOH) on a slide with a coverslip allows for nonfungal cells and debris to be cleared and makes fungal elements more easily visible. KOH-prepared slides can be stained with Calcofluor-white stain and viewed under a fluorescent microscope. Fungal elements are detected by fluorescing on a black background in a blue-white or bright-green color, depending on the microscope filters used. India ink is added to centrifuged sediment of CSF samples for the rapid detection of *C. neoformans*. If present, encapsulated *C. neoformans* buds will appear on a black background with a large clear area around them. Filamentous and branching *Nocardia* species can be differentiated from other actinomycetes with the acid-fast stain. **Gömöri's methenamine silver** stain aids in the detection of *P. jiroveci* by staining carbohydrates in the organisms' cell walls black to brown colors.

MICROSCOPIC DETECTION OF CANDIDA

Candida species can be detected under microscopic examination using a variety of methods and stains. Yeast can be observed directly with a light microscope in wet mount or urine sediment samples. The use of KOH reagent will lyse cells and clear excess debris from samples, aiding in the visualization of yeast and fungal elements. Calcofluor-white stain is used to detect yeast species under a UV microscope by fluorescing fungal elements as a bright-white color that is easily visualized. Easily distinguishable from bacteria, *Candida* presents on a Gram stain as Gram-positive buds, pseudohyphae, or true hyphae. A culture and biochemical testing of urine and vaginal samples containing *Candida* organisms can be used to determine the specific species of yeast responsible for the infection.

POTASSIUM HYDROXIDE (KOH) REAGENT

Potassium hydroxide (**KOH**) reagent is used to aid in the direct examination of yeast and fungal elements present in samples, including, but not limited to, vaginal discharge, skin, hair, and nails. Presence of fungal elements upon visualization aids in the diagnosis and treatment process of suspected fungal infections.

The 10–20% KOH reagent that is added to specimens clears debris and breaks down keratin in hair and nail samples. The breakdown of keratin and the clearing of other debris allows for fungal elements to be more readily observed with a light microscope on a clean glass slide.

KOH procedure:

1. Place the specimen on a clean glass slide — use clean forceps for hair/skin/nail or roll a swab with vaginal discharge/wound sample onto the slide.
2. Add one drop of KOH reagent to the sample on the slide.
3. Place a glass coverslip over the area of the slide; press gently to reduce the presence of bubbles.
4. Place the slide on the microscope stage and examine on low (10×) power to visualize the presence of any fungal structures, such as hyphae or budding yeast.
5. If fungal structures are observed, examine the slide at 40× magnification for further identification and verification of fungi.

CALCOFLUOR-WHITE STAIN

Calcofluor-white is a nonspecific chemifluorescent stain that binds to the cellulose and chitin in cell walls of fungal and parasitic organisms, allowing for visualization via a fluorescent microscope. KOH may be added to the white stain to clear the sample of debris and allow for better visualization. With this method, chitin-containing structures will fluoresce white on a dark background with ultraviolet (UV) light. Evans blue is used as a counterstain to create a dark field, and it allows cells and tissues to be fluoresced and visualized under blue light. Fungal and parasitic elements will fluoresce a bright apple-green color, and all of the other elements will fluoresce at a red-orange color for differentiation between them.

Calcofluor-white procedure:

1. Place the specimen on a clean glass slide.
2. Add one drop of calcofluor-white stain and one drop of KOH (optional) to the slide.
3. Place a glass coverslip over the slide, and press gently to reduce the presence of bubbles.
4. Let the specimen stain, and stain for 1 minute.
5. Examine under UV light at 100× to 400× magnification for the presence of yeast, fungi, or parasitic elements.

TYPES OF FUNGAL MEDIA

Medium	Description
Brain heart infusion agar with blood (BHIB)	Grows most varieties of fungi, especially on sterile human body sites; composed of brain heart infusion and sheep's blood
Sabouraud brain heart infusion agar (SABHI)	Grows most varieties of fungi, and will also grow bacteria
Dermatophyte test medium (DTM)	Good for growing dermatophytes, or skin fungi; antibiotics within the substance obstruct bacterial growth and aid in the development of specific fungi
Cornmeal tween 80	Differential agar used to distinguish varieties of *Candida*
Birdseed agar	Differential agar used to grow *Cryptococcus neoformans*
Potato dextrose agar	Differential agar used to enhance pigmentation of the fungus *Trichophyton rubrum*
Cottonseed agar	Differential agar used to speed the transition from mold to yeast in the fungi *Blastomyces dermatitidis*

MANUAL AND AUTOMATED IDENTIFICATION METHODS

Major yeast and fungus pathogens are differentiated from one another based on their specific biochemical reactions. Biochemical reactions for the identification of pathogens can be performed manually by microbiologists, or they can be performed by sophisticated automated systems. Automated systems are able to differentiate and identify organisms by performing various biochemical reactions on a single test card or panel. A solution is prepared with sterile liquid and an organism inoculated from a culture plate. The inoculate dilution is added to the test card, which has differentiating chemicals loaded into individual test wells. Automated systems compare the pattern of biochemical reactions produced by an isolate to a computerized database for proper identification of the organism. Some organisms may be identified by automated systems within 4 hours; however, most isolates are determined within 12 to 24 hours.

Certain biochemical reactions provide a simple technique for the differentiation of major yeast pathogens. For example, the urease test is a quick biochemical reaction that can determine the difference between the most common, and most easily treatable, yeast pathogen, *C. albicans*, and a less common, potentially fatal, yeast species, *C. neoformans*.

COLONY MORPHOLOGY AND GROWTH CHARACTERISTICS OF MAJOR PATHOGENS

Sabouraud dextrose agar (SDA) is the culture media used for the cultivation of yeasts and molds with a pH of 5.6 to optimize the growth of fungal pathogens. Antibiotics can be added to the medium to inhibit bacterial overgrowth. Due to the slow-growing nature of many fungi, mycological cultures are often kept for four to six weeks to properly assess growth. Listed below are the major human mycological pathogens, with their growth requirements and colony morphology:

C. albicans

- SDA: cream-colored, smooth colonies with a yeast-like odor after 24–48 hours of incubation at 25–37 °C
- Blood agar: white, creamy colonies with foot-like projections around the margin
- CHROMagar: green-colored colonies

C. neoformans

- SDA: white to cream-colored, smooth, mucoid colonies after 48–72 hours of incubation at 37 °C in 5% CO_2
- Bird seed agar: brown-pigmented colonies

A. fumigatus

- SDA: blue-green, velvety or powdery colonies with a narrow white margin on the front of the medium and a pale-yellow color on the back of the medium after 72 hours of incubation at 25–45 °C

H. capsulatum

- SDA: white, fluffy mold within five days of incubation at 25–37 °C. Colonies turn a buff to brown color as they age. Incubation at 37 °C may produce cream-colored, wrinkled, moist, yeast-like colonies.

KERATITIS

Keratitis is inflammation or lesion of the cornea, causing pain, problems with sight, blindness, or other eye damage. Keratitis can occur after injury to the eye, and can either be deep or superficial in nature. Superficial keratitis does not leave a scar on the cornea; however, deep keratitis does tend to leave a scar on the cornea, and this can have a permanent effect on the patient's vision. Fungal keratitis is caused by the fungus *Fusarium*, which is prevalent in plants and soils. It also is a plant pathogen, in addition to the effects it has on human health. The doctor will provide you with corneal scrapings to determine the presence of *Fusarium* in a case of suspected fungal keratitis. Stain the sample and culture it on Sabouraud's agar.

COLONY OF ASPERGILLUS

The fungi *Aspergillus* will grow within 48 hours on a SABHI culture, with the colonies being granular, fluffy, or powdery, and of various colors. *Aspergillus flavus* colonies are brown and green, with a brownish red reverse color; *Aspergillus terreus* colonies are yellow or green, with a yellow reverse color; *Aspergillus fumigatus* colonies are gray or green, with a beige reverse color; and *Aspergillus niger* colonies are yellow or black, with a yellow reverse color. This fungus is responsible for aspergillosis, which can damage the respiratory system, skin, heart, and central nervous system.

Urinalysis and Body Fluids

General Knowledge

URINALYSIS TERMINOLOGY

Prerenal	Classification of kidney disorders caused by problems outside of (before) the kidney, such as inadequate blood flow.
Suprapubic	Above the pubic bone, often the place where suprapubic catheters are placed, especially in males requiring long-term catheterization.
Glycosuria	Presence of glucose in the urine.
Renal threshold	The concentration at which the kidneys begin to remove a substance from the blood and into the urine.
Ascites	Accumulation of serous fluid in the abdominal cavity.
Tamm-Horsfall protein	AKA uromodulin, the most common protein found in normal urine.
Myoglobin	Protein found in muscle tissue.
Amniocentesis	Transabdominal sampling of amniotic fluid from the amniotic sac for prenatal diagnoses of chromosomal disorders and infections.
Pass-through	Duration of time that a drug needs to pass-through the liver and/or kidney.
Osmolality	Concentration of a substance (blood/urine).
Xanthochromic	Yellow-colored, usually in reference to cerebrospinal fluid that has the appearance of urine.
Anuria	Almost no urine discharge, usually due to renal failure or other kidney damage.
Oliguria	Sharp decrease in urine discharge; typically caused by diarrhea, vomiting, perspiration, or other forms of dehydration.
Polyuria	Sharp increase in urine discharge, to a level over 3 L per day; often caused by ingestion of diuretics, caffeine, alcohol, or by diabetes insipidus or mellitus.
Nocturia	Nocturnal increase in urine discharge; often caused by a reduction in bladder capacity due to increased ingestion of fluids, pregnancy, or enlargement of the prostate gland.

AMNIOTIC FLUID MEASUREMENTS

The **lecithin/sphingomyelin ratio** in the amniotic fluid is a good indicator for the lung maturity of the fetus. Via amniocentesis, a sample of surfactant in the amniotic fluid is removed. The lecithin/sphingomyelin ratio is then calculated. If the ratio is less than 2, then the fetal lungs are not producing enough surfactant, and this is an indicator that the fetal lungs may be immature (wet). Determining the lecithin/sphingomyelin ratio is very important because it can help predict and/or prevent fetal respiratory distress after birth.

The **concentrations of creatinine and urea nitrogen** in amniotic fluid are useful for helping determine if amniotic fluid is contaminated with any maternal urine. Using amniocentesis, a sample of amniotic fluid is extracted from the mother's uterus. Because creatinine and urea nitrogen concentrations in the mother's urine are much greater (on the order of ten to fifty times greater) than those concentrations in amniotic fluid, an unexpected high concentration of creatinine and/or

84

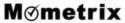

urea nitrogen in the amniotic fluid can indicate contamination of the amniotic fluid with maternal urine, often by bladder puncture.

TYPES OF URINE COLLECTION

Glucose tolerance test	Used to diagnose diabetes or to monitor a diabetic; urine collection every hour, for three hours
Void/Random Sample	Patient collects his or her own urine
Midstream clean catch	Patient cleans pubic area and then collects sample in mid-urination
24-hour	All urine output is collected over a 24-hour period
Suprapubic aspiration	A needle is placed into the bladder and urine is extracted
Two-hour postprandial	Urine is collected two hours after a meal; often performed to measure levels of sugar

Urinalysis Procedures

PHYSICAL AND CHEMICAL PROPERTIES OF URINE

Color	Pale yellow/ amber and darkens when urine is concentrated or other substances (such as blood or bile) or present.
Appearance	Clear but may be slightly cloudy.
Odor	Slight. Bacteria may give urine a foul smell, depending upon the organism. Some foods, such as asparagus, change odor.
Specific gravity	1.015 to 1.025. May increase if protein levels increase or if there is fever, vomiting, or dehydration.
pH	Usually ranges between 4.5 and 8, with average of 5 to 6.
Sediment	Red cell casts from acute infections, broad casts from kidney disorders, and white cell casts from pyelonephritis. Leukocytes >10/ml^3 are present with urinary tract infections.
Glucose, ketones, protein, blood, bilirubin, and nitrate	Negative. Urine glucose may increase with infection (with normal blood glucose). Frank blood may be caused by some parasites and diseases but also by drugs, smoking, excessive exercise, and menstrual fluids. Increased red blood cells may result from lower urinary tract infections.
Urobilinogen	0.1-1.0 units. Increased in liver disease.

ABNORMAL URINE COLORATIONS

Color	Common Causes
Red	Blood, red blood cells, hemoglobin, myoglobin caused by muscle trauma
Dark yellow or amber	Dehydration, infection, fever, or liver problems like hepatitis
Bright yellow or orange	Increased bilirubin, or by medications such as Pyridium, which is used to treat urinary tract infections
Green	Presence of biliverdin, which is introduced by the breakdown of hemoglobin
Black or gray	Presence of melanin or homogentisic acid resulting from a metabolic disorder

IMPORTANCE OF SPECIFIC GRAVITY IN URINALYSIS

Every urinalysis includes a measure of specific gravity, which indicates the degree to which the kidneys can reabsorb water and essential chemicals from the glomerular filtrate. Most kidney disorders impair this function immediately. Specific gravity tests also indicate whether hormone abnormalities or dehydration is present. A normal specific gravity will range from 1.001 to 1.035. If the specific gravity is greater than 1.010, it is called **hypersthenuric** urine. If the specific gravity is less than 1.010, it is called **hyposthenuric** urine. If the specific gravity is exactly 1.010, it is called **isosthenuric** urine.

REFRACTOMETER

Refractometers are used to measure fluid concentration by assessing light refraction through a prism. Refractometers vary in size and sophistication (simple handheld devices to more complex digital devices), so procedures may vary. Generally, the instrument is calibrated with water before the sample is tested. Testing:

1. Turn on equipment.
2. Clean prism with cotton ball and ethanol or according to manufacturer's guidelines.
3. Place sample on prism or in sample well and secure prism.
4. Look through the eyepiece, adjust as needed for manual equipment.
5. Read results expressed in Brix (1 degree Brix = 1 g sucrose in 100 g solution), refractive index (degree to which the light is bent), and/or specific gravity. Digital equipment provides a read-out. Note: Tables are available that provide the refractive index for most common materials

Refractometers may be used to assess urine specific gravity, serum copper sulfate, and serum protein. Sample temperature must be maintained within a prescribed temperature range for some types of refractometers.

BENEDICT'S TEST

Benedict's test is a laboratory test that is used to determine the presence of reducing substances in a urine sample. Some reducing substances that can be present in urine include glucose (which can be indicative of diabetes), other reducing sugars such as lactose and galactose, creatinine, uric acid, or ascorbic acid. The test can tell a technician or a doctor if reducing substances are present in the urine sample, but the test itself is nonspecific. In other words, the test cannot determine the specific reducing substance present. To perform the test, Benedict's reagent (a solution of copper sulfate, sodium carbonate, and sodium citrate) is added to a urine sample, and the mixture is heated. A red, yellow, or orange precipitate is indicative of the presence of a reducing substance in the urine. The precipitate is formed because the copper sulfate in the Benedict's reagent is reduced by any reducing substance contained in the urine.

URINALYSIS PROCEDURES

Test	Procedure
pH	Insert indicator paper or reagent strip into urine, remove excess, wait time according to manufacturer's guidelines, and compare to color chart.
Glucose	Use reagent strip OR place 5 mL of Benedict solution in test tube and 8 drops of urine, and mix. Boil solution for 2 minutes with Bunsen burner or spirit lamp with tube at about 45° angle or place tube in boiling water for 5 minutes. Cool tube and check color for amount of glucose with blue equal to 1+ and orange/red, 4+.
Nitrate/ Nitrite	Enzymes produced by bacteria change nitrate into nitrite, which is measured as an indirect method to detect UTI. Urine must have been in bladder for at least 4 hours, so first morning sample is usually used. Dip reagent strip in the urine sample and read results at 30 to 60 seconds and match against color chart with positive findings indicated by change to light to dark pink.

Test	Procedure
Bilirubin	Protect urine specimen from light and examine when fresh. Dip reagent strip in urine and read test results at 30 to 60 seconds and match against color chart with colors ranging from buff (1+) to tan/purple (3+) for positive reaction OR use Ictotest®.
Urobilinogen	Test fresh specimen between 2 and 4 PM (peak levels), especially for liver function testing. Dip reagent strip in the urine sample, read results at 30 to 60 seconds, and match to color chart with positive color changes ranging from peach-colored (0.2 mg/dL) to bright pink (8 mg/dL).
Protein	Use reagent strip OR place 5 mL of urine in a test tube and add 2 drops of sulfosalicylic acid. Observe for formation of white precipitate and as negative or from + to ++++ (trace to large amount) depending on the amount of precipitate.
Ketones	Use Acetest® tablets OR dip ketone stick in urine, wait 15 seconds, and monitor color changes. Positive changes are light lavender (5 mg/dL) to purple (160 mg/dL).
Blood	Place 12 mL urine in conical tube, centrifuge 5 minutes (medium speed), pour off supernatant, shake tube, use pipette to remove 1 drop of sediment and place on slide for microscopic examination. RBCs appear colored (yellow/green).
Leukocyte esterase	Obtain clean catch urine sample in sterile container, dip reagent strip into urine and check color chart after 2 minutes. No color change is negative but shades of pink to purple indicate trace to large amounts.

REAGENT STRIPS

Lab technicians use reagent strips to examine the chemical composition of a urine sample. The following chemicals can be assessed: bilirubin, glucose, nitrite, blood, protein, white blood cells, ketones, and urobilinogen. Also, reagent strips can determine the specific gravity and pH of urine. These strips work as follows: they are dipped into the urine sample and change colors depending on the composition of the urine. As long as basic restrictions regarding room temperature and procedure are followed, these reagent strips are highly accurate.

CONFIRMATORY URINE TESTS

Test	Procedure
Clinitest®	Confirms the presence of glucose in the urine. Drop alkaline copper reagent tables in a tube containing 5 drops of urine and 10 drops of distilled water, which will boil. Wait 15 seconds after boiling stops, gently shake tube, and check color against chart. Blue is negative and colors from green to orange indicate the presence of 1/4% (+) to 2% (++++) glucose.
Ictotest®	Confirms the presence of bilirubin in the urine. Place 10 drops of urine on a special absorbant mat, place a reagent table in the middle of the moistened are and then one drop of distilled water on the tablet. After 5 seconds, place another drop of distilled water on the table. Wait 60 seconds and observe the color about and under the tablet. Blue or purple color indicates the presence of bilirubin.
Acetest® (Acetone test)	Confirms the presence of ketones in the urine. Place tablet on clean dry white paper and place 1 drop of urine on top of tablet. Wait 30 seconds and check color against color chart. No change in color is negative and shades of lavender (light, medium, and dark) indicate small, moderate, and large amounts of ketones.

Test	Procedure
Sulfosalicylic acid (SSA)	Confirms the presence of protein in the urine. If urine is cloudy, centrifuge before test. Fill tube (10×75 mm) one-third full of urine and add one-third tube of 3% SSA solution. Cover with paraffin film/cap and mix by inverting. Check results by holding in front of lined/text test strip. If the lines/text are clear, the result is negative, slightly cloudy but lines/text visible, 1+; lines are visible but unable to read text, 2+; no lines/text visible, 3+; totally opaque/gelled, 4+.

ADDIS COUNT PROCEDURE

The Addis count is a laboratory technique to calculate the number of formed elements in a urine sample. The formed elements include blood cells (white blood cells and red blood cells) and casts. In this test, a 12-hour urine specimen is collected. Formalin is used as a preservative for the urine sample. After the 12-hour period, a specified quantity of the urine specimen is put in a centrifuge. Part of any resuspended urine sediment is then placed into a Neubauer blood-counting chamber. The squares of the blood-counting chamber are then examined. Any formed elements, such as casts, white blood cells, or red blood cells, that are present are counted. The total number of formed elements in the entire urine sample is then calculated. This test can be used on the urine of patients that have kidney disease.

URINE MICROSCOPY
CASTS

Cast	Indication
White blood cells	Infection or inflammation
Red blood cells (appear brown or yellow)	Renal disease
Hyaline	Renal disease, heart failure, or glomerulonephritis. Often seen after stress, excessive exercise, or dehydration.

CRYSTALS

Crystal	Appearance
Cystine	Colorless, hexagonal plates
Tyrosine	Yellow or colorless thin needles
Cholesterol	Clear, flat rectangular crystals
Uric acid	Various; colorless or yellow, and shaped as cubes, diamonds, plates, or needles
Bilirubin	Yellow to brown plates, granules, or needles
Calcium oxalate	Various; dumbbell, octahedral, or envelope shapes
Leucine	Yellow to brown spheres, often with striations

ALKALINE CRYSTALS

Alkaline Crystal	Appearance
Triple phosphate	Triangular or hexagonal prisms, similar to a coffin shape
Calcium phosphate	Crystals may be irregularly-shaped and large, or in granular sheets or plates
Amorphous phosphate	Colorless granules
Ammonium biurate	Brown or yellow, with striations; may contain irregular projections
Calcium carbonate	Small and colorless, often dumbbell-shaped

TERMS FOR ABNORMAL URINE

Myoglobinuria: Condition in which urine contains myoglobin; often the result of muscle trauma, coma, or muscle destruction

Hematuria: Condition in which urine contains intact red blood cells; often caused by renal tumors, menstruation, or pregnancy

Hemoglobinuria: Condition in which urine contains hemoglobin; often caused by infections, transfusion reactions, hemolytic anemia, or burns

Ketonuria: Condition in which urine contains ketones; often the result of diabetes mellitus, dehydration, or chronic imbalance electrolytes

Bilirubinuria: Condition in which urine contains bilirubin; often caused by liver disease, hepatitis, or cirrhosis of the liver

MAPLE SYRUP URINE DISEASE

Individuals with the genetic metabolic disorder known as maple syrup urine disease have a natural deficiency of branched-chain keto acid decarboxylase, resulting in a diminished metabolism of valine, leucine, and isoleucine. The condition gets its name from the aroma emanating from the urine, breath, and skin of infants with the condition. This condition is most common in the Amish and Mennonite communities, and can be identified with a Guthrie bacterial inhibition test. If it is not treated, it can lead to intellectual disability, hypoglycemia, convulsions, and even death.

Special Tests

QUALITATIVE AND QUANTITATIVE TEST METHODS FOR DETERMINING THE PRESENCE OF FECAL FAT

There are both qualitative and quantitative means of identifying malabsorbed fat in feces. The quantitative method involves collecting stool samples over a period of 72 hours, mixing the samples, and analyzing a small sample. The level of fats in the sample can be measured through the process known as saponification. The qualitative method of measuring fecal fat is to take a random stool sample and combine it with a fat-soluble stain on a microscope slide. Sudan III, Sudan IV, Nile Blue, and Oil Red O are all used for this purpose. Malabsorbed fecal fat will present as reddish orange oil bubbles.

TYPES OF FECAL MATTER

Type/Consistency	Indication
Watery	Diarrhea
Ribbon-like	Bowel obstruction
Black/tarry	Bleeding in the gastrointestinal tract
Frothy, bulky, or yellow colored	Malabsorption syndrome, in which stool contains too much fat
Containing mucus	Colitis or inflammation of the intestinal wall

REINSCH'S TEST

The Reinsch's Test is a laboratory test used to determine the presence of heavy metals in a sample, often urine. In this particular test, the urine sample is dissolved in a solution of hydrochloric acid (HCl). After the urine is dissolved, a strip of copper is placed into the solution. If a heavy metal is present, the copper strip will develop a colored coating. A silver coating may indicate the presence

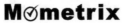

of mercury, while a blackish/blue color (or another dark color) may indicate the presence of another heavy metal, such as antimony, arsenic, bismuth, selenium, or thallium. The test is a rapid one, and is good for a quick, initial screening. However, the findings of this test should be confirmed with other laboratory techniques.

TRINDER REACTION

The Trinder Reaction is used most often to determine the presence of salicylate in the urine. A solution containing ferric chloride is added to the urine sample in question. An iron complex will form between the ferric chloride and the salicylate, if salicylate is present. This reaction will turn the solution a purple color. The test is very rapid, and this is one of its positive points. However, the test has the possibility for false positive results as well. A purple color will also be produced if any enol or phenol is present in the urine, as well as if the patient has an elevated urine bilirubin level of 1 mg/dL or greater.

HCG HEMAGGLUTINATION INHIBITION TEST

The HCG hemagglutination test is used to determine pregnancy by examining a urine sample. Add a sample of urine to two drops of HCG antiserum. To this, add red blood cells that have been coated in HCG. If HCG is present in the urine sample, the HCG antiserum binds to the HCG present, therefore making it impossible for the HCG antiserum to react with the red blood cells coated in HCG. This leads to the red cells not agglutinating, and a donut shape consisting of red blood cells will form. This donut shape indicates HCG in the urine sample. However, if there is no HCG present in the urine sample, the HCG antiserum will bind with the HCG coated red blood cells. No donut pattern of red blood cells will form. Instead, there will be a diffuse pattern of red blood cells. This diffuse pattern indicates that no HCG is present in the urine sample. The patient is not pregnant, or is pregnant more than six months.

MANUAL TESTING

Test	Procedure
Bilirubin	Uncoagulated blood sample allowed to clot at room temperature and then centrifuged and supernatant separated immediately for examination. <u>Direct</u>: Dilute sample by mixing 1 mL with 4 mL saline. Label 2 tubes for direct bilirubin (DB) and serum blank (SB). Place 1 mL diluted serum and 2 mL 0.05 hydrochloric acid in each tube. Place 0.5 mL Diazo II reagent in DB and in exactly 60 seconds add 0.1 mL ascorbic acid, mix, and add 1.5 mL alkaline tartrate and read color results in 5-10 minutes. To tube SB, place 0.5 mL Diazo I reagent, 0.5 mL ascorbic acid, and 1.5 mL alkaline tartrate, and mix to use as serum blank.
Occult blood (gastric)	Sample is applied to paper reagent strip coated with guaiac, which changes color to blue in the presence of blood within 1 minute. The sample may also be applied to a slide (thin smear), which is examined microscopically.

BODY FLUID CYTOCENTRIFUGATION

Cytocentrifugation ("cytospin") uses a special centrifuge with slide holders that have attached funnels to hold body fluid that has been mixed with a medium in prescribed amounts. The process is able to concentrate cells that occur in small numbers in a sample. During centrifugation (usually at about 500 rpm for about 5 minutes), the fluid is wicked into a filter and onto a slide in a thin monolayer. Albumin (11% or 22%) may be added to serous fluids to preserve morphology as centrifugation may result in some distortion (although clumping patterns and ratio of nucleus to cytoplasm are unchanged). Albumin should not be added to synovial fluid. Cells in body fluids are

90

similar to those in peripheral blood, and morphology is similar but counts are usually less. Once the slide is prepared, staining may be done to facilitate evaluation.

SEMEN ANALYSIS

Before his semen may be collected for an infertility analysis, and a male must be abstinent for three days. Such a waiting period is not necessary before other laboratory tests. Semen is collected in a sterile container and cannot be obtained in the presence of condoms or spermicides. Semen is collected and stored at room temperature.

These are the parameters for a semen analysis:

Color and clarity	grayish-white and translucent
pH	7.3-7.8
Viscosity (1–4)	1
Volume	2–5 mL
Coagulation and liquefaction	~30 minutes after collection
Sperm motility	>60%
Forward progression of sperm	>50%
Count	>40 million
Normal morphology (no double or deformed tails or heads)	>30%

Practice Test

Want to take this practice test in an online interactive format?
Check out the bonus page, which includes interactive practice questions and
much more: **mometrix.com/bonus948/mlsamt**

1. Receiving cannot accept a specimen unless it has

    a.   A correct, legible label

    b.   An uncontaminated, signed requisition with billing information

    c.   An intact container with correct media

    d.   All of the above

2. A laboratory refrigerator used to store volatile, flammable liquids can hold

    a.   120 gallons of class I, II, and IIIA liquids

    b.   180 gallons of class I, II, and IIIA liquids

    c.   200 gallons of class I, II, and IIIA liquids

    d.   50 gallons of class I, II, and IIIA liquids

3. Disease incidence predicts

    a.   How probable it is a patient will develop a disease, and its etiology

    b.   How likely a test result is to be right or wrong, given certain variables

    c.   How likely the patient with a negative test really does not have the condition

    d.   How likely the patient with a positive test result really has the condition

4. Beer's law in spectrophotometry

    a.   Means a transparent sample transmits 0% light

    b.   Only applies if absorbance is between 0.1 and 1.0

    c.   Means an opaque sample transmits 100% light

    d.   Uses a visible spectrum from 340 nm to 500 nm

5. Naming bacteria by looking at their size and shape under the microscope, and the colony morphology on media is

    a.   Differential identification

    b.   Numeric taxonomy

    c.   Presumptive identification

    d.   TaqMan electrophoresis

6. The hospital department that studies alcohol, drugs, poisons, and heavy metals is

    a.   Serology/Immunology

    b.   Toxicology

    c.   Cytology

    d.   Endocrinology

7. A hemoglobin electrophoresis result of adult hemoglobin (HbA) or HbA2 means the patient has

a. Sickle cell anemia
b. Fetal hemoglobin
c. Normal hemoglobin
d. Hemolytic anemia

8. US law overrides the patient's right to confidentiality if

a. The patient has a sexually transmitted disease or tuberculosis (TB).
b. The caregiver is likely to be infected.
c. Authorities suspect child abuse or neglect under CAPTA.
d. All of the above

9. The recall rate is also known as the

a. Sensitivity
b. Specificity
c. Aliquot
d. Circadian rhythm

10. Biochemistry usually requires

a. Lavender, light blue, and black blood collection tubes
b. Red, pink, and yellow blood collection tubes
c. Green, gray, and marbled serum-separator tube (SST) blood collection tubes
d. Navy, purple, and brown blood collection tubes

11. A normal kidney function study shows a

a. BUN to creatinine ratio between 15:1 and 20:1
b. Alkaline phosphatase 30 to 85 international milliunits/mL
c. Serum aspartate aminotransferase 5 to 40 international units/L
d. Amylase 56 to 190 international units/L

12. A newborn's jaundice could be caused by

a. Erythroblastosis fetalis
b. Kernicterus
c. Physiologic jaundice from poor fluid intake
d. All of the above

13. Lipids from carbohydrate and alcohol sources are

a. Anions
b. Triglycerides
c. Cholesterol
d. Eluent

14. When serum proteins indicate disease, the doctor usually follows up with

a. Total protein, albumin, and globulin
b. Ascites
c. Protein electrophoresis
d. Bilirubin

15. Elevated creatine phosphokinase (CPK) could mean myocardial infarction, but could also mean

a. Alcoholism, hypothyroidism, cardioversion, or clofibrate use
b. Aspirin, burns, warfarin, or sickle cell anemia
c. Lung disease or congestive heart failure
d. Crushing injury, bowel infarction, or opiate use

16. A patient whose cortisol level is high at both 8:00 AM and 4:00 PM likely has

a. Addison's disease
b. Natriuretic factor
c. Diabetes insipidus
d. Cushing syndrome

17. Decreased sodium in the blood is

a. Hypernatremia, often from diabetes, burns, or Cushing syndrome
b. Hyponatremia, often from vomiting and diarrhea, furosemide, or Addison's disease
c. Hyperkalemia, often from acidosis, spironolactone, or kidney failure
d. Hypokalemia, often from alkalosis, stomach cancer, or eating too much licorice

18. CPK in a patient with a myocardial infarction will

a. Rise 6 hours after heart attack, peak in 18 hours, and return to baseline in 3 days
b. Rise 6 to 10 hours after heart attack, peak at 12 to 48 hours, and return to baseline in 4 days
c. Rise 24 to 72 hours after heart attack, peak in 4 days, and return to baseline in 14 days
d. Cause a corresponding rise in alpha-fetoprotein

19. The panic value for blood pH is

a. 7.35
b. Less than 7.20
c. 80 to 100 torr
d. 4.0 to 8.0 mcg/L

20. When performing a sweat test for cystic fibrosis, the MT ensures

a. The current never exceeds 4 mA for 5 min and 25 volts.
b. The current is 10 mA for 30 min and 10 volts.
c. The current does not pass the patient's trunk.
d. Both a and c are correct

21. If the doctor suspects the patient has Hodgkin's disease, then the correct stain for the smear is

a. Periodic acid-Schiff (PAS)
b. Sudan black B (SBB)
c. Leukocyte alkaline phosphatase (LAP)
d. Lactophenol cotton blue (LPCB)

22. A battlement scan is preferable to a wedge scan for studying bone marrow because

a. Battlement technique distributes cells evenly across the slide.
b. Lymphocytes concentrate in the feather.
c. Wedge technique causes leukocytes to pool in different sections of the slide.
d. Both a and c

23. A bleeding patient with a coagulation deficiency needs

a. 225 mL of fresh frozen plasma at +18°C
b. 15 mL of cryoprecipitate at +18°C
c. 300 mL of platelet pheresis at +20°C
d. 520 mL of whole blood at +4°C

24. Confirm a fungal infection found through microscopy with a

a. Latex serology for cryptococcal antigen
b. Fungal serology titer of more than 1:32 that increases x4 or more 3 weeks later
c. Complement fixation for coccidiomycosis and histoplasmosis
d. Immunodiffusion for blastomycosis.

25. Two modern flocculation tests that replace the older Venereal Disease Research Laboratory (VDRL) test for syphilis screening are

a. Plasmacrit test (PCT) and rapid plasma reagin (RPR) test
b. Fluorescent treponemal antibody absorption (FTA-ABS) and enzyme-linked immunosorbent assay (ELISA)
c. Treponemal-specific microhemagglutination (MHA-TP) and T. pallidum particle agglutination test (TP-PA)
d. Captia Syphilis-G enzyme immunoassay (EIA) and cold agglutinins

26. To make a dilution of ½ or 1:2

a. Dilute ½ mL of serum with 2 mL of saline
b. Dilute 1 mL of serum with 2 mL of saline
c. Test undiluted serum for antibody/antigen reaction against a control
d. Dilute 1 mL of serum with 1 mL of saline

27. A Monospot test uses ingredients from

a. Guinea pig, cow, and horse
b. Sheep, pig, and horse
c. Dog, sheep, and rabbit
d. Fish, cat, and ferret

28. A prozone phenomenon occurs when performing an antibody titer on a patient with

a. Epstein-Barr virus (EBV)
b. Raynaud disease
c. Both syphilis and HIV
d. Immunoglobulin G (IgG) antibodies

29. An Rh- mother who is pregnant with the child of an Rh+ father needs Rh immunoglobulin (RhoGAM)

a. Even if the pregnancy ends in miscarriage or abortion
b. At 6 to 28 weeks of pregnancy and again within 72 hours after her delivery.
c. During her labor
d. Both a and b

30. If a patient has a mild transfusion reaction

    a. Eosinophilia, hypocalcemia, leukopenia, and pancytopenia may occur.
    b. Dyscrasia, leukocytosis, hypercalcemia, and leukemia may occur.
    c. Anemia, hypokalemia, glycosuria, and pancytopenia may occur.
    d. Hemolysis, hyperkalemia, hypoglycemia, and hemoglobinuria may occur.

31. Type O blood has

    a. B antigen and anti-A antibody
    b. A antigen and anti-B antibody
    c. No A or B antigens and both anti-A and anti-B antibodies
    d. Both A and B antigens and no anti-A or anti-B antibodies

32. Choose the top priority transfusion patient from the following list.

    a. Cardiac surgery patient who lost more than 1,200 mL of blood
    b. Trauma patient with a hemoglobin of 5 g/dL
    c. Pernicious anemia patient
    d. Hemophiliac boy at regular clinic visit

33. Reject a transfusion request when

    a. Recipient blood specimen is hemolyzed.
    b. The patient armband does not have a unique identifier.
    c. Donor blood is lipemic, clotted, or contains foreign objects.
    d. All of the above

34. The continuous recording thermometer in a Blood Bank refrigerator must be set at

    a. +4°C
    b. 0°C
    c. +6°C
    d. -5°C

35. If the surgical team suspects the patient may suffer blood loss greater than 500 mL, they order

    a. Fresh frozen plasma
    b. Whole blood
    c. Factor VIII
    d. Packed red blood cells

36. When blood typing by hemagglutination, the last O-shape is in the #64 incubation well, before the blood becomes solid red dots. Report the titer as

    a. 1:128
    b. 1:64
    c. 1:1024
    d. 1:512

37. When using an automatic pipette to perform immunoassays, the laboratory must have a procedure in place to detect

a. Assay signal response
b. Target analytes
c. Sensitivity validation
d. Carryover effects

38. When gamma and scintillation counters are used for radioimmunoassay (RIA), each day the technologist must

a. Calibrate, record the results, and compare them to the previous day's values
b. Test the background radioactivity in multiwell counters only
c. Lengthen the counting times for quantitative procedures to improve validity
d. Decontaminate sinks and benches monthly

39. To diagnose a urinary tract infection correctly, the microbiology lab requires a

a. Midstream urine collection (MSU)
b. Witnessed urine collection
c. 24-hour urine collection
d. Random urine collection

40. When assisting the doctor with cerebrospinal fluid (CSF) collection, you need 4 tubes for

a. Cell count, glucose and protein, gram stain and culture, virology/mycology/cytology.
b. Immunoelectrophoresis
c. Fungus, oncology, and SMA-12
d. Neutrophilia, lymphocytophilia, glutamine, and lactate dehydrogenase (LDH)

41. Fusobacteria cause

a. Botulism and Listeria infections
b. Lyme disease and Helicobacter pylori stomach ulcers
c. Pyorrhea and Lemierre syndrome
d. Chlamydial genital infections and pneumonia

42. The type of media required to incubate a TB culture correctly is

a. Tinsdale
b. Sheep blood agar
c. Modified Wadowsky-Yee (MWY)
d. Löwenstein-Jensen (LJ) egg

43. To find parasites under the microscope, set the magnification to

a. 40x
b. 10x
c. 1,000x
d. 400x

44. Identify the parasite that must be reported to Public Health authorities

a. Crypto (Cryptosporidium parvum)
b. Hookworm (Ancylostoma duodenale)
c. Tapeworm (Cestoda)
d. Pinworm (Enterobius)

45. To identify motile trophozoites

a. Examine blood smears and blood antigens
b. Perform a string test
c. Use Snap n' Stain on sputum
d. Wet mount fresh, liquid stool with LPCB stain

46. Public Health requires you to keep positive parasitology samples preserved for

a. The patient's lifetime
b. One year
c. Ten years
d. One month

47. Shine a Wood's lamp over the patient's skin to help you collect

a. Malaria specimens
b. Public Health specimens
c. Toxicology specimens
d. Mycology specimens

48. When the doctor orders acid-fast stain to detect TB, the technologist

a. Looks for red bacteria under the oil-immersion lens
b. Lyzes the cells by holding them in a Bunsen burner flame 30 seconds
c. Pours 1% methylene blue stain into the LJ egg plate
d. Decolorizes the bacteria with acetone and water solution

49. Normal urinary output for a 24-hour urine test is

a. 4 quarts
b. 150 to 500 mL
c. 30 L
d. 750 to 2,000 mL

50. Urate crystals found during microscopic urinalysis indicate

a. Urea-splitting bacteria are present
b. Poisoning
c. Gout
d. Hyperparathyroidism

Answer Key and Explanations

Question	Question	Question	Question	Question
1. D	11. A	21. C	31. C	41. C
2. A	12. D	22. D	32. B	42. D
3. A	13. B	23. A	33. D	43. B
4. B	14. C	24. B	34. A	44. A
5. C	15. A	25. A	35. A	45. D
6. B	16. D	26. D	36. B	46. B
7. C	17. B	27. A	37. D	47. D
8. D	18. A	28. C	38. A	48. A
9. A	19. B	29. D	39. A	49. D
10. C	20. D	30. A	40. A	50. C

Answer Explanations

1. D: Receiving cannot accession a specimen without

- A label that clearly states the patient's name, collection date, doctor's name and contact information, specimen type, and test required.
- An uncontaminated, valid requisition bearing the doctor's signature, patient's billing information, and pertinent information (acute or convalescent phase, antibiotic use, fever, or traveler).
- Intact specimen container.
- Correct media type or preservative used for the specimen type.
- Same-day collection date, or preincubated at room temperature or subcultivated, and then vented, to prevent false-negatives of nonfermentative species.

If the specimen does not meet these conditions, call the doctor's office and get the missing information. Discard the specimen if you cannot obtain full information, and inform the doctor's office that recollection is required.

2. A: Class IA, IB, and IC are flammables. Class II, IIIA, and IIIB are combustibles. No more than 120 gallons of class I, II, and IIIA liquids can be stored in a lab fridge, and, of those, no more than 60 gallons may be class I and II. Do not locate more than three storage cabinets in one fire area. No more than 50% of the flammables can be stored for teaching. Use DOT-approved glass, metal, or polyethylene containers no larger than 1.1 gallons (4 liters).

3. A: Because disease incidence measures how prevalent a disease is among a given population in a specific place, over a specific time. Incidence predicts how probable it is a patient will develop a disease, and its etiology (likely cause). B,C, and D are incorrect because they refer to a related concept called predicted values, which estimate how likely a test result is to be right or wrong, given certain variables such as the patient's age, occupation, race, income, how long the symptoms have lasted, and if there is fever.

4. B: Because Beer's law states absorbance is proportional to the concentration of a solution, but Beer's law only applies if absorbance is between 0.1 and 1.0. Different substances absorb different light wavelengths, so a spectrophotometer (Spec-20) compares the intensity of light entering a sample and exiting from it (percent transmittance) to find the concentration of the sample. A completely transparent sample has 100% transmittance. A completely opaque sample has 0% transmittance. Visible spectrum light ranges from 440 nm to 700 nm.

5. C: Note the color, outline (circular, rhizoid, or wavy), elevation (convex, flat, or raised), and translucency (opaque, translucent, or transparent) for presumptive identification. Differential identification means naming bacteria according to their headspace gases and volatile compounds they release as they grow on media, with a spectrometer (microDMx). Adanson's numerical taxonomy (phonetics) ranks microorganisms according to how similar they are genetically and morphologically. Closely related bacteria form a cluster, which is classified into objective, repeatable taxa. TaqMan, SWOrRD, and MicroSeq are quick screening kits. They are not as accurate as cultures but are quicker when time is critical. Polymerase chain reaction (PCR) in quick kits amplifies the genetic material, and then the 1450 base pair region of the 16S rDNA gene is sequenced by electrophoresis.

6. B: Serology/Immunology studies antibodies in the liquid part of blood. Cytology studies cells for cancer, such as Pap smears. Endocrinology studies hormones, such as diabetes and acromegaly.

7. C: Hemoglobin electrophoresis differentiates hemoglobin into normal HbA and normal HbA2, or abnormal HbS in sickle cell patients, or HbC in hemolytic anemia patients, or HbF in a fetus or newborn.

8. D: Doctors, nurses, social workers, chiropractors, law officers, daycare staff, clergy, teachers, and psychologists were declared mandatory reporters in 1996. This means they must report certain occurrences or suspicions orally to the proper authorities within 24 hours and follow up with a written report within 48 hours. For example, a doctor must report STD or TB to Public Health to prevent an epidemic. Caregivers have the right to know the patient's diagnosis if it puts them at risk for infection or assault. Suspicion of child abuse, exploitation, or neglect is reported to Child Protective Services under the Child Abuse Prevention and Treatment Act (CAPTA). Each state has an abuse hotline. Many states require anyone who has reasonable cause to report child or elder abuse or face civil liability. You must know the law of the state in which you practice.

9. A: Sensitivity (recall rate) measures how many times a test produces true-positive results, which indicates a patient probably has a disease, compared with the gold standard test for that particular illness. Sensitivity allows early detection of disease and prevents epidemics. Divide the number of patients who definitely have the disease and test positive by the total patients tested who have the disease (including those who tested false-negative), and multiply by 100 to obtain the percentage sensitivity. Specificity measures how many times a test produces true-negative results, meaning patients probably do not have a disease, compared with the gold standard test for that particular illness. Specificity is important for cancer chemotherapy and other toxic treatments. Aliquot is dividing a solution into equal parts. Aliquot allows very expensive reagents or drugs, and blood samples that are below scale, to be used efficiently. Circadian rhythm is a normal daily flow that affects hormones, which are normally higher in the morning than in the afternoon.

10. C: Hematology requires mostly lavender, light blue, and black tubes. Blood Bank and Public Health require red, pink, and yellow tubes. Toxicology requires navy, purple, and brown tubes. If you draw the wrong color tube, it contains an inappropriate anticoagulant, and the test will be invalidated.

11. A: Blood urea nitrogen (BUN) and creatinine are waste products of protein metabolism, measured in kidney function tests performed with a 24-hour urine. If the kidneys do not filter properly, creatinine output in the urine decreases, and creatine blood levels increase. High creatinine (more than 1.5 mg/dL) and BUN (more than 20 mg/dL) means the patient has a kidney disease (e.g., glomerulonephritis, pyelonephritis, stones, tubular necrosis, tumors). BUN and creatinine must be in correct proportion for optimal health. ALP and AST are liver function tests. Amylase is a pancreas test.

12. D: Newborn jaundice is different from adult jaundice. Babies have more red blood cells and reticulocytes than adults do. Babies have immature livers that are not yet efficient at breaking down bilirubin. Adult jaundice is usually from hepatitis or cirrhosis of the liver. Erythroblastosis fetalis means the baby's Rh factor is incompatible with his mother's Rh, leading to hemolytic disease of the newborn. Kernicterus means the bilirubin is greater than 5 mg/dL, resulting in hemolytic anemia if not treated with phototherapy (blue lights). Physiologic jaundice occurs in breastfed babies released from the hospital too early and without a vitamin K injection, but resolves in a week with adequate fluids.

13. B: Anions are negatively charged ions of chloride and bicarbonate. Cholesterol is lipids from animal sources that climb after a fatty meal. An eluent is a solvent used for chromatography.

14. C: The serum proteins test includes total protein, albumin, and globulin. Ascites is swelling of the abdomen from extra fluid in the peritoneum, resulting from end-stage diseases of the heart, kidney, liver, ovary, and pancreas. When serum proteins make the doctor suspect one of these diseases, the doctor follows up with protein electrophoresis. Four globulin fractionations are added to the total protein and albumin alpha-1 globulin, alpha-2 globulin, beta globulin, and gamma globulin. Electrophoresis patterns and the patient's history of drug use help pinpoint the diagnosis, which may extend to rheumatoid arthritis, muscle tumors, and immune deficiencies. Bilirubin is the brownish-red bile pigment from broken down blood cells in the liver.

15. A: Cardiac enzymes elevate soon after a heart attack, but that is not the only possible root cause. CPK elevates in alcoholism; cardiac catheterization; stroke; clofibrate use; electric shock applied during resuscitation; low thyroid hormone and high thyroid stimulating hormone; and after surgery. B and D refer to situations that cause AST enzyme to rise. C refers to situations that cause LDH enzyme to rise.

16. D: Cortisol is an adrenal stress hormone that is normally higher around 800 in the morning (6 to 28 mcg/dL) and lower at 400 in the afternoon (2 to 12 mcg/dL). The fluctuation is a normal diurnal variation. Cushing syndrome patients have sustained high cortisol. Addison's disease patients have chronically low cortisol levels, diagnosed by a 24-hour urine test for 17-hydroxycorticosteroids. Abnormal cortisol levels also appear in thyroid and pituitary gland disease, obesity, and cancer, and when steroids, diuretics, or birth control pills are used, but it is not the same pattern as Cushing syndrome. B refers to atrial natriuretic factor (ANF), produced by the heart's atria during volume overload and high blood pressure.

17. B: Hyponatremia results from too much water and not enough salt in the bloodstream. Hyponatremia often presents as a urine sample with a specific gravity (SG) lower than the normal 1.015 to 1.025 and closer to the SG of water (1.000). Hypernatremia refers to too much salt in the bloodstream, which increases SG above 1.025. Hyperkalemia and hypokalemia refer to the level of potassium, not sodium.

18. A: CPK is the first enzyme to rise following a heart attack, so doctors measure it before the other cardiac enzymes. If creatine kinase-MB (CK-MB) rises, it means the heart sustained severe damage. B refers to the response of AST to a heart attack. C refers to the response of LDH to a heart attack. D does not apply because alpha-fetoprotein (AFP) is used to find liver disease, testicular cancer, and birth defects.

19. B: pH stands for percentage of hydrogen. A blood pH test is performed with arterial blood gasses to determine if the patient has acidosis or alkalosis. The blood must be kept in a narrow range of pH from 7.35 to 7.45, so answer A would be low normal. Answer C, 80 to 100 torr, refers to normal percentage of oxygen. D is incorrect because an abnormal PSA result for prostate cancer is unrelated to blood pH.

20. D: When performing a sweat test for cystic fibrosis, the technologist must avoid burning the patient or causing depolarization of the heart. The technologist uses only a battery-powered iontophoretic current and it cannot exceed 4 mA for 5 minutes. The technologist uses only the patient's arm or leg for sweat collection and ensures the electrodes do not cross over the patient's trunk. The technologist never performs iontophoresis near an open oxygen source, but asks the nurse to give the patient a face mask or nasal cannula during the test.

21. C: Hematologists use LAP stain to highlight neutrophils when the patient has many white blood cells but not leukemia (leukemic reaction). Microbiologists use periodic acid-Schiff (PAS) to stain carbohydrates, collagen, fibrin, and mucin purple. Sudan black B (SBB) is specifically for acute leukemia patients; it helps to differentiate between immature cells by staining lipids in myeloid leukemia that are absent in lymphoid leukemia. LPCB is mixed with 10% potassium hydroxide (KOH) to identify fungus.

22. D: Make a bone marrow slide with a battlement technique so the review is standardized, with even cell distribution. Wedge push technique (feathered end) causes the white cells to pool unevenly on the slide. On the side edges and in the feather of a wedge push slide, concentrated pockets of eosinophils, monocytes, and segmented neutrophils will be found. Small lymphocytes concentrate in the center of the slide.

23. A: Fresh frozen plasma can be used for a bleeding patient with a coagulation deficiency, or a trauma patient who needs additional red blood cells. Reserve whole blood for the resuscitation of trauma victims. Cryoprecipitate is appropriate for hemophiliacs, von Willebrand disease, and hypofibrinogenemia. Platelet pheresis is useful for patients with thrombocytopenia or platelet dysfunction.

24. B: First, gently scrape suspected fungus off the patient's skin. Mix two drops of 10% potassium hydroxide (KOH) and one drop of LPCB on a glass slide, cover it, and warm it to observe budding yeasts. Add a drop of calcofluor white before warming to see fluorescent infected tissue. Put a drop of India ink on a wet mount to see clear cryptococcal capsules. Confirm the microscopic exam with fungal serology when you test the skin scraping and again in three weeks. The doctor may follow up by ordering latex serology for cryptococcal antigen to find meningitis, complement fixation for coccidiomycosis and histoplasmosis, and immunodiffusion for blastomycosis.

25. A: The old screening test for syphilis is VDRL, which measures Treponema pallidum antibodies by flocculation reaction to the diphosphatidyl glycerol in ox heart extract. However, VDRL misses cases of syphilis that are less than four weeks old, and half of cases that are in the late stages. VDRL is not very sensitive, and often gives a false-positive result for patients with the following conditions pregnancy, hepatitis, HIV, leprosy, lupus (SLE), Lyme disease, malaria, mononucleosis, pneumonia, rheumatic fever, or rheumatoid arthritis. PCT and RCR are less likely to be confounded, and since they require less blood, are replacing VDRL. ELISA confirms syphilis infection by identifying the specific antibodies. FTA-ABS is 100% accurate for secondary syphilis, but it is expensive, and the patient will always test positive once infected. Captia is required to confirm RPR. Cold agglutinins increase in children with congenital syphilis.

26. D: You must know how to dilute to perform a titer, which measures how many times a blood sample must be diluted with saline before an antibody can no longer be found in it.

First, check the antibody/antigen reaction against the controls with undiluted serum. To prevent blood clotting (rouleaux formation) during dilution, warm the blood and saline to body temperature (37°C) for 10 minutes before diluting. Dilute 1 mL of serum with 1 mL of saline for a dilution of ½, or 12. Pipette off 1 mL of this dilution into an aliquot tube. Add 1 mL of saline, and it becomes a 14 dilution. If you dilute up to 132 and get no reaction, the end-point titer is 16.

27. A: Monospot heterophile antibodies test confirms an early infection of mononucleosis, caused by Epstein-Barr virus. If the infection is older than 9 weeks, then the doctor orders EBV antibody test. On a glass slide, mix a drop of the patient's blood with guinea pig kidney antigen to absorb Forssman antibodies. Add beef red blood stroma to absorb non-Forssman antibodies. Mix with horse blood. Guinea pig agglutination means the patient has early mononucleosis. Beef should not agglutinate. Monospot can be false-negative on children younger than 10, or before two weeks of infection. B, C, and D are not applicable to Monospot.

28. C: Patients coinfected with HIV and syphilis are immunosuppressed. When performing a titer to find antibodies in an HIV/syphilitic, beware prozone phenomenon. The coinfected patient's undiluted serum may produce a false-negative result because it does not agglutinate. Alternatively, it may show very little agglutination at low dilutions, but agglutinates more at higher dilutions because of excess antibodies. Monospot is used to find EBV mononucleosis. Reynaud disease is characterized by rouleaux formation and high cold agglutinin titers. IgG occurs in patients who are convalescing from mononucleosis.

29. D: RhoGAM is the brand name for Rh immunoglobulin. It is administered to Rh- women who acquired anti-D antibodies from a previous blood transfusion or pregnancy. The infant and father do not receive RhoGAM at all. If there is a live birth, the mother gets 300 mcg of RhoGAM during week 26 to 28 of her pregnancy, and again before her infant is 3 days old. If the pregnancy miscarries before week 13 or is aborted, then the mother gets a lower dose of 50 mcg of MICRhoGAM. If the miscarriage or abortion happens after week 13, use RhoGAM.

30. A: The first lab sign of a mild transfusion reaction is the oxyhemoglobin dissociation curve shifts left. Later, the number of eosinophils will increase and the calcium level will drop. Finally, white blood cells will decrease, and then all blood cells will decrease. Minimize the chance of transfusion reaction by washing the donor's red blood cells in sterile normal saline before transfusion. If the doctor anticipates a mild transfusion reaction, he/she may give antihistamines to the patient before transfusion, and may order the removal of white cells from the bag of blood by a Sepacell R-500 leukocyte reduction filter. Irradiated blood products prevent fatal transfusion-associated graft-versus-host disease (TA-GVHD). The safest way for a patient to prepare for elective surgery is to bank his own blood for transfusion (autologous donation).

31. C: No A or B antigens and both anti-A and anti-B antibodies. Type O- blood is the universal donor because it has no A or B antigens, or Rh+ antibodies. If there is no time to crossmatch a trauma patient, then O- blood is given without compatibility testing to prevent death. A routine type and cross takes 45 minutes and the delay could be fatal.

32. B: Blood Bank triages patients in the following priority sequence (1) emergency trauma victims with isovolemic anemia from hemorrhage; (2) surgical patients who lose more than 3 cups of blood; (3) regular users of coagulation factors. If you anticipate a blood shortage because of a massive trauma, then contact the nurse manager as soon as possible. The surgical team may decide to cancel elective surgery, or delay it until the patient is medically treated to reduce anemia. If surgery must proceed, the surgical team may consider the following blood conservation methods if you warn them ahead of time erythropoietin, autologous donations, or hemodilution before surgery; cell savers, hypotension, electrocautery, and lasers during surgery; and administration of antifibrinolytics after surgery.

33. D: A type and cross is very time-consuming (45 minutes) and must meet very specific safety standards to avoid a transfusion reaction. All of the following conditions must be met

- Specimens labeled at the patient's bedside with full name or the emergency department identification number; initials are unacceptable. Specimens must not have pink serum. Donor blood must not be clotted, fatty, or contaminated.

- Patient wears an identification band, which is checked at collection and transfusion times. The band must not be taped to the bed. The patient's name and a unique identification number (Blood Bank identification number, hospital number, health insurance number, or unique lifetime identifier) must appear on the band, in case there is a patient with a similar name.
- Requisitions must bear the collector's and identifier's names, collection date and time (in case antibodies develop), the ordering doctor's name, the amount and type of blood requested, the patient's date of birth (if known), relevant patient history (e.g., pregnant and bleeding; signs of transfusion reaction).

34. A: Other laboratory refrigerators can safely range from 0 °C to +6 °C. However, Blood Bank must keep blood products at a stable +4 °C to ensure their safety. Only freezers should be in the minus degrees range, as ice crystals forming in the blood would render it useless and potentially fatal if transfused.

35. D: The surgical team carefully reviews the patient's pre-op blood work to anticipate any complications that might occur in the operating room. An anesthetized patient whose heart rate increases during surgery, or whose blood pressure drops, can quickly lose 1.5 liters of blood. Initially, the surgical team will want packed red blood cells standing by from Blood Bank. The nurses weigh the patient and count the number of saturated pads in the theater to help the surgeon and anesthetist calculate blood loss. A 2x2 gauze pad holds 5 mL of blood and a 4x4 gauze pad holds 12 mL of blood. If the blood loss approaches 500 mL, the surgeon orders a transfusion. Although plasma volume increases after blood loss, red cell volume does not return to normal for several weeks without compensation from a transfusion. Whole blood may be required to ensure recovery is as quick and painless as possible.

36. B: Blood typing (A, B, O) to prevent blood transfusion reactions is usually performed by hemagglutination. Antibodies crosslink red blood cells coated with antigen. Nonagglutinated blood forms a solid red dot at the bottom of an incubation well. Agglutinated blood appears diffuse or O-shaped at the bottom of an incubation well. The technologist makes serial dilutions of serum in incubation wells and measures the highest dilution still capable of agglutinating the blood. Most agglutination reactions occur in less than 2 minutes. Label the control wells Neg and Pos. Label the remaining incubation wells 2, 4, 8, 16, 32, 64, 128, 256, 512, and 1024 for the serial dilutions. Look along the row of wells for the last O-shape before the blood becomes solid red dots. If the last O is at 64, then report the titer as 1:64.

37. D: If the laboratory's immunoassay setup includes an automatic pipette, then the lab manager must create a procedure to determine if carryover effects are contaminating the samples. The most common procedure requires running known high samples first, followed by known low samples. If the results of the low-level material are affected, then carryover is present. The procedure must define the benchmark below which low-level samples are affected. Quality Assurance must review the results of each analytical run to ensure there are no results exceeding the benchmark. The procedure then states what the technologist must do with the subsequent samples. Usually, the technologist is expected to repeat the subsequent samples, using a clean pipette for each.

38. A: The technologist must determine if the machines are performing to the standard with daily radioisotope calibrations that are recorded for accreditation purposes. Sinks and benches are decontaminated daily, not monthly. If the lab uses or stores radionuclides in excess of those found in commercial 125-I RIA kits, then the Nuclear Regulatory Commission requires the technologist to be familiar with the radiation manual, which covers safe shielding, storage, decontamination, counting, disposal, and reporting procedures.

39. A: MSU is required to diagnose cystitis and pyelitis accurately. Witnessed collection is only required for drug testing. 24-hour urines are for hormone tests. Random urine may have contamination, so while it is suitable for chemistry, random urine is inaccurate for microbiology. Collect midstream urine any time of day, in a sterile, lidded container. Your microbiologist may want the patient to use a benzalkonium chloride wipe before collection. Without a wipe, the sample is not a clean catch. Do not touch the inside of the container, as it contaminates the specimen and produces a false-positive.

40. A: Only a physician can collect cerebrospinal fluid (CSF) from a lumbar puncture. The medical technologist just prepares a collection tray and assists as ordered. The tray must contain the following iodine prep; alcohol prep; 3 cc of 1% lidocaine; 25g, 5/8" needle; 22g, 1.5" needle; atraumatic spinal needle (to prevent postcollection headache); syringe; four sterile red stoppered tubes; 4x4 gauze; sponge forceps; sterile towels; small basin; and a Band-Aid. The physician collects the fluid between L3 and L4 in the patient's spine and hands you the tubes. Label one tube each for cell count, glucose and protein, gram stain and culture, and virology/mycology/cytology. You only need a fifth tube if the physician wants globulin immunoelectrophoresis, which is rare. C and D tests are included in A, and it is unnecessary to requisition them separately.

41. C: The pathogenic phyla are xenobacteria, cyanobacteria, firmicutes, flavobacteria, fusobacteria, planctomycetes, proteobacteria, spirochaetes, and verrucomicrobia. Planctomycetes causes chlamydia and pneumonia. Spirochaetes cause Lyme disease. Proteobacteria causes stomach ulcers. Firmicutes cause food poisoning. Fusobacteria cause pockets of pus in the gums that can break off into septic blood clots in the jugular vein of the neck. The septic clots can travel to cause abscesses in distant parts of the body, such as the brain, joints, kidney, and liver. Lemierre syndrome from gum disease was common until the discovery of antibiotics.

42. D: Tuberculosis is a fussy bacterium to grow in the lab and requires egg media. Tinsdale is used to find C. diphtheria. Sheep blood is used to find slow-growing anaerobic bacteria. MYW is used to find Legionella pneumonia. It is important for the medical technologist to know what type of infection the doctor suspects, so the correct media can be used for culture. Failure to pick the correct media may result in a false-negative and the disease will go undiagnosed.

43. B: To find parasites such as worms, set the microscope's magnification to 10x. Parasites often cause bleeding, so set the microscope to 40x to find the blood cells. Higher powers are unnecessary to view animal parasites and count cells, and would just slow down the medical technologist's slide reading. Calibrate the ocular micrometer every time a new technologist is hired, each time you change optics, and annually thereafter.

44. A: In the United States, the medical technologist is required by law to report the following nine parasites to Public Health authorities if they are found in patient samples Cryptosporidium parvum, Cyclospora cayetanensis, Entamoeba histolytica, hematoxylin, Giardia duodenalis, Plasmodium falciparum, Taenia, Trichinella spiralis, and Enterobius vermicularis. Hookworm, tapeworm, and pinworm are very common infestations and do not need to be reported. Your lab must provide reference slides or a parasite atlas for you to compare against the patients' specimens. Keep positive specimens in your lab for at least one year, either as a permanently stained slide, or as a preserved stool sample that is safely stored. Public Health may order them for examination.

45. D: Giardia lamblia is a parasite that lives in the small intestine of humans who consume contaminated food or water. Giardia causes traveler's diarrhea. Giardia cysts are activated by stomach acid and become trophozoites. The medical technologist can get the patient to swallow a string for several hours and then examine it for trophozoites, but many patients are uncooperative and prefer to leave a stool sample instead. To prepare the wet mount, strain well-formed stool. Concentrate it in the centrifuge at 2000 rpm for 4 minutes in a conical tube. Ream the tube with a wooden stick. Add 10% formalin. Make a tan suspension. You should be able to read a newspaper through the slide. Examine microscopically at 10x for parasites and 40x for blood. Use an ocular micrometer to measure parasites. Mix stool with PVA plastic powder to glue it onto the slide before permanent staining with iodine or Snap n' Stain.

46. B: Parasites are a serious Public Health issue. It is important to prevent parasites acquired in foreign countries from spreading through the American populace. Even though you check your patient's specimen against reference slides or a parasite atlas, you could miss rare species or misidentify the parasite in its different stages of development. A Public Health official has the right to check your slide for one year after initial testing. To ensure your test is accurate, use positive and negative controls to check your antigens every time you receive a new shipment and every month thereafter. Use the right stain for the right specimen. Refrigerate stool within three hours of receiving it, if you do not have time to fix it with preservative.

47. D: The medical technologist uses a Wood's lamp to help identify fungus on the patient's skin before collecting it. Fungus will fluoresce bright lime green under the Wood's light, so the medical technologist will find it easily and can scrape it off with a tongue depressor into a sterile container for testing. Malaria parasites are found in blood smears. Public Health specimens are usually blood serology or stool for parasites. Toxicology specimens are usually red, navy, or purple stoppered blood tubes for drugs or heavy metals.

48. A: The technologist submerges the TB smear for five minutes in Kinyoun carbol fuchsin stain, decolorizes with a 70% ethanol/0.5% hydrochloric acid solution, followed by 1% methylene blue stain for 1 minute. Tubercle bacteria appear red under the oil-immersion lens. Do not hold the slide in the flame. It lyzes the cells by cooking them. If the slide feels too hot when placed on the back of your hand, then heat killed the TB bacteria. Do not overwash with water, and do not use acetone to decolorize.

49. D: A patient should produce at least 500 mL (2 cups) of urine every day. Ideally, a patient should produce 750 mL (3 cups) to 2,000 mL (5 cups) of urine to maintain good health. If the patient has vomiting and diarrhea, or an enlarged prostate gland or severe infection, or uses too much medication, then he will produce scanty urine (oliguria). Some of the drug overdoses that decrease urinary output are anticholinergics, methotrexate, and diuretics. Patients whose kidneys are failing have anuria, which strictly interpreted means absence of urine, but they actually produce 100 mL or less of urine per day. Patients who have diabetes insipidus or diabetes mellitus often produce far too much urine (3½ quarts or more). They are very thirsty and may drink more than a gallon of fluid per day (more than 12 glasses). The antidepressant lithium is one drug that can cause frequent urination as an adverse effect.

50. C: Patients with gout have extreme pain in their great toes due to needles of uric acid crystals that form around their joints. Patients with struvite crystals in their urine have bacterial infections. Patients with tyrosine or cystine crystals in their urine may be poisoned or have a serious metabolic disorder. Patients with phosphate or calcium oxalate crystals in their urine have too much parathyroid hormone or malabsorption. Crystals do not appear in healthy urine.

How to Overcome Test Anxiety

Just the thought of taking a test is enough to make most people a little nervous. A test is an important event that can have a long-term impact on your future, so it's important to take it seriously and it's natural to feel anxious about performing well. But just because anxiety is normal, that doesn't mean that it's helpful in test taking, or that you should simply accept it as part of your life. Anxiety can have a variety of effects. These effects can be mild, like making you feel slightly nervous, or severe, like blocking your ability to focus or remember even a simple detail.

If you experience test anxiety—whether severe or mild—it's important to know how to beat it. To discover this, first you need to understand what causes test anxiety.

Causes of Test Anxiety

While we often think of anxiety as an uncontrollable emotional state, it can actually be caused by simple, practical things. One of the most common causes of test anxiety is that a person does not feel adequately prepared for their test. This feeling can be the result of many different issues such as poor study habits or lack of organization, but the most common culprit is time management. Starting to study too late, failing to organize your study time to cover all of the material, or being distracted while you study will mean that you're not well prepared for the test. This may lead to cramming the night before, which will cause you to be physically and mentally exhausted for the test. Poor time management also contributes to feelings of stress, fear, and hopelessness as you realize you are not well prepared but don't know what to do about it.

Other times, test anxiety is not related to your preparation for the test but comes from unresolved fear. This may be a past failure on a test, or poor performance on tests in general. It may come from comparing yourself to others who seem to be performing better or from the stress of living up to expectations. Anxiety may be driven by fears of the future—how failure on this test would affect your educational and career goals. These fears are often completely irrational, but they can still negatively impact your test performance.

Elements of Test Anxiety

As mentioned earlier, test anxiety is considered to be an emotional state, but it has physical and mental components as well. Sometimes you may not even realize that you are suffering from test anxiety until you notice the physical symptoms. These can include trembling hands, rapid heartbeat, sweating, nausea, and tense muscles. Extreme anxiety may lead to fainting or vomiting. Obviously, any of these symptoms can have a negative impact on testing. It is important to recognize them as soon as they begin to occur so that you can address the problem before it damages your performance.

The mental components of test anxiety include trouble focusing and inability to remember learned information. During a test, your mind is on high alert, which can help you recall information and stay focused for an extended period of time. However, anxiety interferes with your mind's natural processes, causing you to blank out, even on the questions you know well. The strain of testing during anxiety makes it difficult to stay focused, especially on a test that may take several hours. Extreme anxiety can take a huge mental toll, making it difficult not only to recall test information but even to understand the test questions or pull your thoughts together.

Effects of Test Anxiety

Test anxiety is like a disease—if left untreated, it will get progressively worse. Anxiety leads to poor performance, and this reinforces the feelings of fear and failure, which in turn lead to poor performances on subsequent tests. It can grow from a mild nervousness to a crippling condition. If allowed to progress, test anxiety can have a big impact on your schooling, and consequently on your future.

Test anxiety can spread to other parts of your life. Anxiety on tests can become anxiety in any stressful situation, and blanking on a test can turn into panicking in a job situation. But fortunately, you don't have to let anxiety rule your testing and determine your grades. There are a number of relatively simple steps you can take to move past anxiety and function normally on a test and in the rest of life.

Physical Steps for Beating Test Anxiety

While test anxiety is a serious problem, the good news is that it can be overcome. It doesn't have to control your ability to think and remember information. While it may take time, you can begin taking steps today to beat anxiety.

Just as your first hint that you may be struggling with anxiety comes from the physical symptoms, the first step to treating it is also physical. Rest is crucial for having a clear, strong mind. If you are tired, it is much easier to give in to anxiety. But if you establish good sleep habits, your body and mind will be ready to perform optimally, without the strain of exhaustion. Additionally, sleeping well helps you to retain information better, so you're more likely to recall the answers when you see the test questions.

Getting good sleep means more than going to bed on time. It's important to allow your brain time to relax. Take study breaks from time to time so it doesn't get overworked, and don't study right before bed. Take time to rest your mind before trying to rest your body, or you may find it difficult to fall asleep.

Along with sleep, other aspects of physical health are important in preparing for a test. Good nutrition is vital for good brain function. Sugary foods and drinks may give a burst of energy but this burst is followed by a crash, both physically and emotionally. Instead, fuel your body with protein and vitamin-rich foods.

Also, drink plenty of water. Dehydration can lead to headaches and exhaustion, especially if your brain is already under stress from the rigors of the test. Particularly if your test is a long one, drink water during the breaks. And if possible, take an energy-boosting snack to eat between sections.

Along with sleep and diet, a third important part of physical health is exercise. Maintaining a steady workout schedule is helpful, but even taking 5-minute study breaks to walk can help get your blood pumping faster and clear your head. Exercise also releases endorphins, which contribute to a positive feeling and can help combat test anxiety.

When you nurture your physical health, you are also contributing to your mental health. If your body is healthy, your mind is much more likely to be healthy as well. So take time to rest, nourish your body with healthy food and water, and get moving as much as possible. Taking these physical steps will make you stronger and more able to take the mental steps necessary to overcome test anxiety.

Mental Steps for Beating Test Anxiety

Working on the mental side of test anxiety can be more challenging, but as with the physical side, there are clear steps you can take to overcome it. As mentioned earlier, test anxiety often stems from lack of preparation, so the obvious solution is to prepare for the test. Effective studying may be the most important weapon you have for beating test anxiety, but you can and should employ several other mental tools to combat fear.

First, boost your confidence by reminding yourself of past success—tests or projects that you aced. If you're putting as much effort into preparing for this test as you did for those, there's no reason you should expect to fail here. Work hard to prepare; then trust your preparation.

Second, surround yourself with encouraging people. It can be helpful to find a study group, but be sure that the people you're around will encourage a positive attitude. If you spend time with others who are anxious or cynical, this will only contribute to your own anxiety. Look for others who are motivated to study hard from a desire to succeed, not from a fear of failure.

Third, reward yourself. A test is physically and mentally tiring, even without anxiety, and it can be helpful to have something to look forward to. Plan an activity following the test, regardless of the outcome, such as going to a movie or getting ice cream.

When you are taking the test, if you find yourself beginning to feel anxious, remind yourself that you know the material. Visualize successfully completing the test. Then take a few deep, relaxing breaths and return to it. Work through the questions carefully but with confidence, knowing that you are capable of succeeding.

Developing a healthy mental approach to test taking will also aid in other areas of life. Test anxiety affects more than just the actual test—it can be damaging to your mental health and even contribute to depression. It's important to beat test anxiety before it becomes a problem for more than testing.

Study Strategy

Being prepared for the test is necessary to combat anxiety, but what does being prepared look like? You may study for hours on end and still not feel prepared. What you need is a strategy for test prep. The next few pages outline our recommended steps to help you plan out and conquer the challenge of preparation.

STEP 1: SCOPE OUT THE TEST

Learn everything you can about the format (multiple choice, essay, etc.) and what will be on the test. Gather any study materials, course outlines, or sample exams that may be available. Not only will this help you to prepare, but knowing what to expect can help to alleviate test anxiety.

STEP 2: MAP OUT THE MATERIAL

Look through the textbook or study guide and make note of how many chapters or sections it has. Then divide these over the time you have. For example, if a book has 15 chapters and you have five days to study, you need to cover three chapters each day. Even better, if you have the time, leave an extra day at the end for overall review after you have gone through the material in depth.

If time is limited, you may need to prioritize the material. Look through it and make note of which sections you think you already have a good grasp on, and which need review. While you are studying, skim quickly through the familiar sections and take more time on the challenging parts.

Write out your plan so you don't get lost as you go. Having a written plan also helps you feel more in control of the study, so anxiety is less likely to arise from feeling overwhelmed at the amount to cover.

STEP 3: GATHER YOUR TOOLS

Decide what study method works best for you. Do you prefer to highlight in the book as you study and then go back over the highlighted portions? Or do you type out notes of the important information? Or is it helpful to make flashcards that you can carry with you? Assemble the pens, index cards, highlighters, post-it notes, and any other materials you may need so you won't be distracted by getting up to find things while you study.

If you're having a hard time retaining the information or organizing your notes, experiment with different methods. For example, try color-coding by subject with colored pens, highlighters, or post-it notes. If you learn better by hearing, try recording yourself reading your notes so you can listen while in the car, working out, or simply sitting at your desk. Ask a friend to quiz you from your flashcards, or try teaching someone the material to solidify it in your mind.

STEP 4: CREATE YOUR ENVIRONMENT

It's important to avoid distractions while you study. This includes both the obvious distractions like visitors and the subtle distractions like an uncomfortable chair (or a too-comfortable couch that makes you want to fall asleep). Set up the best study environment possible: good lighting and a comfortable work area. If background music helps you focus, you may want to turn it on, but otherwise keep the room quiet. If you are using a computer to take notes, be sure you don't have any other windows open, especially applications like social media, games, or anything else that could distract you. Silence your phone and turn off notifications. Be sure to keep water close by so you stay hydrated while you study (but avoid unhealthy drinks and snacks).

Also, take into account the best time of day to study. Are you freshest first thing in the morning? Try to set aside some time then to work through the material. Is your mind clearer in the afternoon or evening? Schedule your study session then. Another method is to study at the same time of day that you will take the test, so that your brain gets used to working on the material at that time and will be ready to focus at test time.

STEP 5: STUDY!

Once you have done all the study preparation, it's time to settle into the actual studying. Sit down, take a few moments to settle your mind so you can focus, and begin to follow your study plan. Don't give in to distractions or let yourself procrastinate. This is your time to prepare so you'll be ready to fearlessly approach the test. Make the most of the time and stay focused.

Of course, you don't want to burn out. If you study too long you may find that you're not retaining the information very well. Take regular study breaks. For example, taking five minutes out of every hour to walk briskly, breathing deeply and swinging your arms, can help your mind stay fresh.

As you get to the end of each chapter or section, it's a good idea to do a quick review. Remind yourself of what you learned and work on any difficult parts. When you feel that you've mastered the material, move on to the next part. At the end of your study session, briefly skim through your notes again.

But while review is helpful, cramming last minute is NOT. If at all possible, work ahead so that you won't need to fit all your study into the last day. Cramming overloads your brain with more information than it can process and retain, and your tired mind may struggle to recall even previously learned information when it is overwhelmed with last-minute study. Also, the urgent nature of cramming and the stress placed on your brain contribute to anxiety. You'll be more likely to go to the test feeling unprepared and having trouble thinking clearly.

So don't cram, and don't stay up late before the test, even just to review your notes at a leisurely pace. Your brain needs rest more than it needs to go over the information again. In fact, plan to finish your studies by noon or early afternoon the day before the test. Give your brain the rest of the day to relax or focus on other things, and get a good night's sleep. Then you will be fresh for the test and better able to recall what you've studied.

STEP 6: TAKE A PRACTICE TEST

Many courses offer sample tests, either online or in the study materials. This is an excellent resource to check whether you have mastered the material, as well as to prepare for the test format and environment.

Check the test format ahead of time: the number of questions, the type (multiple choice, free response, etc.), and the time limit. Then create a plan for working through them. For example, if you have 30 minutes to take a 60-question test, your limit is 30 seconds per question. Spend less time on the questions you know well so that you can take more time on the difficult ones.

If you have time to take several practice tests, take the first one open book, with no time limit. Work through the questions at your own pace and make sure you fully understand them. Gradually work up to taking a test under test conditions: sit at a desk with all study materials put away and set a timer. Pace yourself to make sure you finish the test with time to spare and go back to check your answers if you have time.

After each test, check your answers. On the questions you missed, be sure you understand why you missed them. Did you misread the question (tests can use tricky wording)? Did you forget the information? Or was it something you hadn't learned? Go back and study any shaky areas that the practice tests reveal.

Taking these tests not only helps with your grade, but also aids in combating test anxiety. If you're already used to the test conditions, you're less likely to worry about it, and working through tests until you're scoring well gives you a confidence boost. Go through the practice tests until you feel comfortable, and then you can go into the test knowing that you're ready for it.

Test Tips

On test day, you should be confident, knowing that you've prepared well and are ready to answer the questions. But aside from preparation, there are several test day strategies you can employ to maximize your performance.

First, as stated before, get a good night's sleep the night before the test (and for several nights before that, if possible). Go into the test with a fresh, alert mind rather than staying up late to study.

Try not to change too much about your normal routine on the day of the test. It's important to eat a nutritious breakfast, but if you normally don't eat breakfast at all, consider eating just a protein bar. If you're a coffee drinker, go ahead and have your normal coffee. Just make sure you time it so that the caffeine doesn't wear off right in the middle of your test. Avoid sugary beverages, and drink enough water to stay hydrated but not so much that you need a restroom break 10 minutes into the test. If your test isn't first thing in the morning, consider going for a walk or doing a light workout before the test to get your blood flowing.

Allow yourself enough time to get ready, and leave for the test with plenty of time to spare so you won't have the anxiety of scrambling to arrive in time. Another reason to be early is to select a good seat. It's helpful to sit away from doors and windows, which can be distracting. Find a good seat, get out your supplies, and settle your mind before the test begins.

When the test begins, start by going over the instructions carefully, even if you already know what to expect. Make sure you avoid any careless mistakes by following the directions.

Then begin working through the questions, pacing yourself as you've practiced. If you're not sure on an answer, don't spend too much time on it, and don't let it shake your confidence. Either skip it and come back later, or eliminate as many wrong answers as possible and guess among the remaining ones. Don't dwell on these questions as you continue—put them out of your mind and focus on what lies ahead.

Be sure to read all of the answer choices, even if you're sure the first one is the right answer. Sometimes you'll find a better one if you keep reading. But don't second-guess yourself if you do immediately know the answer. Your gut instinct is usually right. Don't let test anxiety rob you of the information you know.

If you have time at the end of the test (and if the test format allows), go back and review your answers. Be cautious about changing any, since your first instinct tends to be correct, but make sure you didn't misread any of the questions or accidentally mark the wrong answer choice. Look over any you skipped and make an educated guess.

At the end, leave the test feeling confident. You've done your best, so don't waste time worrying about your performance or wishing you could change anything. Instead, celebrate the successful completion of this test. And finally, use this test to learn how to deal with anxiety even better next time.

> **Review Video: Test Anxiety**
> Visit mometrix.com/academy and enter code: 100340

Important Qualification

Not all anxiety is created equal. If your test anxiety is causing major issues in your life beyond the classroom or testing center, or if you are experiencing troubling physical symptoms related to your anxiety, it may be a sign of a serious physiological or psychological condition. If this sounds like your situation, we strongly encourage you to seek professional help.

Additional Bonus Material

Due to our efforts to try to keep this book to a manageable length, we've created a link that will give you access to all of your additional bonus material:

<u>mometrix.com/bonus948/mlsamt</u>

114